Schizophrenia

Schizophrenia: Science and Practice

EDITED BY **John C. Shershow**

HARVARD UNIVERSITY PRESS

Cambridge, Massachusetts, and London, England   1978

Library of Congress Cataloging in Publication Data
Main entry under title:
Schizophrenia.

    Bibliography: p.
    Includes index.
    CONTENTS: Historical and philosophical perspectives:
Shershow, J. C. Approaches to understanding schizo-
phrenia. Savodnik, I. The manifest and the scientific
images.—Etiology, the nature-nurture interaction:
Kety, S. Heredity and environment. Lidz, T. A develop-
mental theory.—Bioscientific research: Klerman, G. L.
The evolution of a scientific nosology. Creese, I. and
Snyder, S. H. Biochemical investigation. Hollister, L.
Psychopharmacology.—Care and treatment, the
human dimension: Borus, J. F. and Hatow, E.
The patient and the community. Schwartz, D. P.
Psychotherapy. Mosher, L. R. and Menn, A. Z.
The surrogate "family," an alternative to
hospitalization.
    1. Schizophrenia—Addresses, essays, lectures.
I. Shershow, John C. [DNLM: 1. Schizophrenia. WM200.
3 S337]
RC514.S3364   616.8'982   78-6317
ISBN   0-674-79112-6

Preface

The genesis of this book was a series of lectures delivered in the Department of Psychiatry at the Massachusetts General Hospital. During what one might call its epigenesis—the unfolding of its final form—each contributor and I have worked together toward a written narrative that would present many of the complex issues surrounding that group of behaviors and feelings which we refer to as schizophrenia. An important part of this effort is the discussion sections. By posing questions to each contributor to clarify and expand on some of the points raised in the chapter, I have tried to recapture at least a hint of the stimulation and excitement that took place not only following the formal lectures but also in the hallways and around the luncheon table.

A word is necessary about the grammatical use of gender in this book. An attempt has been made to avoid the convention of using the masculine gender except when one is referring specifically and exclusively to women. Unfortunately, in some instances avoiding the practice is quite cumbersome, and at those points I have let stand (although not always comfortably) the *he* or *his* to refer to all persons.

Two important acknowledgments are in order. Roerig, a division of Pfizer Pharmaceuticals, provided generous financial support for the original lecture series and thus very tangibly made possible this undertaking. The staff of Harvard University Press, particularly Eric Wanner and Susan Wallace, worked closely with me, providing invaluable suggestions and encouragement throughout the revision and production of the book.

J.C.S.
March 1978

Contents

Historical and Philosophical Perspectives

1   Approaches to Understanding Schizophrenia   3
    John C. Shershow
2   The Manifest and the Scientific Images   21
    Irwin Savodnik ·

Etiology: The Nature-Nurture Interaction

3   Heredity and Environment   47
    Seymour Kety
4   A Developmental Theory   69
    Theodore Lidz

Bioscientific Research

5   The Evolution of a Scientific Nosology   99
    Gerald L. Klerman
6   Biochemical Investigation   122
    Ian Creese and Solomon H. Snyder
7   Psychopharmacology   152
    Leo Hollister

Care and Treatment: The Human Dimension

8   The Patient and the Community   171
    Jonathan F. Borus and Elaine Hatow
9   Psychotherapy   197
    Daniel P. Schwartz
10   The Surrogate "Family," an Alternative
to Hospitalization   223
    Loren R. Mosher and Alma Z. Menn

Index   241

PART ONE

Historical and Philosophical Perspectives

Approaches to Understanding Schizophrenia

JOHN C. SHERSHOW

When I was a medical student, a pathologist advised our class to remember, as had generations of physicians before us, that "if one knew syphilis, one knew medicine." And indeed, as amply demonstrated in his subsequent lectures, so diverse were the symptoms of this disease, so numerous were its clinical complications, and so varied were the treatments at one time or another proposed that little doubt was left in my mind as to the veracity of this statement. Truly, what case conference is complete that does not mention tertiary syphilis in its differential diagnosis? There was, however, one problem with the maxim, as my mentor pointed out. Because clinicians at that time saw so few cases of syphilis, especially the secondary and tertiary variety, to use this route to learn medicine was perhaps somewhat impractical.

Much later, after I began my psychiatric training, it occurred to me that, analogously, if one knew schizophrenia one would very likely know psychiatry. For so diverse were the symptoms of this disease, so numerous were its clinical complications, and so varied were the treatments at one time or another proposed that little doubt was left in my mind as to the veracity of this second statement! Indeed, one can scarcely imagine a psychiatric case conference in which some participant does not raise the issue, "Is this person schizophrenic?" Certainly, the classic descriptions of schizophrenia, which prior to the current Kraepelinian revival in American psychiatry were predominantly from Eugen Bleuler's traditional text (1924), contain many passages

3

like the following, in which one is cautioned to look for schizophrenia lurking virtually anywhere in the vast array of psychopathology:

> The beginning of schizophrenia is in reality usually furtive. Even though the disease often becomes obvious to the relatives first through an acute attack, a good anamnesis usually reveals certain previous changes of character, or other schizophrenic signs. Whether the inclination to retirement, often noticeable even in childhood, combined with a certain degree of irritability, is an expression of a disposition, or the actual beginning of the disease, cannot be decided. In many cases the disease itself makes itself felt by a gradual decline of acquired skill and of capacity to work; in others, neurasthenic, hysteric, or compulsive neurotic symptoms are for years mistaken for the disease and treated unsuccessfully. [p. 435]

Well, time passes. What had been an ever-present disease, lurking ominously behind even the mildest and least dysfunctional of symptoms, has become a sort of shrinking phantom of psychiatry. The group of individuals with "affective disorders" seems with every monthly issue of the *Archives of General Psychiatry* to incorporate yet another segment of the formerly schizophrenic population. Simultaneously, investigators such as Otto Kernberg (1975) and Heinz Kohut (1974) have pointed out that another large group of persons formerly assumed to be "mildly" or "latently" schizophrenic have, rather, borderline personality organizations or narcissistic personality disorders. And after we make a careful organic assessment of psychotic patients, in search of neurologic diseases such as temporal lobe epilepsy or subacute sclerosing panencephalitis, as well as the large number of drug related, endocrine related, and degenerative diseases, then the list of patients for whom we could confidently write "schizophrenia," as our professional ancestors once did, has surely shrunk mightily. I often think these days, as I used to in studying syphilis in medical school, that I could learn a lot from schizophrenia—if only I could find a case of it!

The point, of course, is that the definition of "schizophrenia" has varied tremendously throughout modern psychiatric history, not to mention the period prior to the modern era. This book reviews much of what is now known about the syndrome, although psychiatrists share no greater unity of view today than did their forebears. The historical survey in this chapter and Dr. Savodnik's philosophic discussion in chapter 2 bring out the diversity of our conceptions of schizophrenia and the degree to which this diversity represents differences on the most basic epistemologic questions. Part two presents two contrasting ideas about the etiology of schizophrenia, and part three recounts the impressive advances that have been made in recent years in the objective and statistical description of the syndrome, its possible biochemical correlates, and pharmacologic treatment. Finally, in part four several dedicated clinicians write of traditional as well as some innovative ways of treating this complex disorder.

I must ask, then, for a certain conceptual forbearance as I discuss some historical trends in the treatment of what I will call, for want of a better general term, "insanity." By insanity I mean to refer to mental illness of psychotic proportions that may be characterized by a single acute episode followed by the return of more or less complete premorbid functioning; or by numerous acute episodes followed by the return of more or less complete functioning between episodes; or by chronic impairment of functioning. Many at the current time will question whether the first two examples truly represent schizophrenia, and will accept only the third type—what is commonly known as "poor prognosis schizophrenia" or "process schizophrenia." Such a view, of course, has varied considerably throughout modern psychiatric history and it is important to bear in mind that many of the differences between our approaches and those of our professional ancestors may reflect this fact.

Further, in my review of these historical themes I will take largely a hospital or inpatient perspective. I do this not merely because my current professional role centers around inpatient treatment, although I grant that this is no small motivation. I do it rather because until a few years ago virtually all significant psychiatric treatment took place in an inpatient setting. An outpatient approach to any disorder, especially a psychotic one, has been a relatively recent innovation. Thus, if my historical review seems to parallel some of the trends in inpatient psychiatry itself, this results not so much from the bias of my perspective as from the way in which the orientation of inpatient psychiatry is historically interlocked with conceptualizations of psychotic illness.

Moral Treatment

This tradition arose at the end of the eighteenth century both from Pinel's work in France and from the simultaneous founding of the York Asylum in England by William Tuke. In America it rapidly spread through the work of such figures as Issac Ray, Pliny Earle, and John Butler and through the founding of moral treatment centers such as the Friends Asylum in Philadelphia, McLean Hospital in Boston, and the Hartford Retreat in Connecticut (see Bockoven 1972; Shershow 1977a).

Moral treatment argued against the treatment of mental illness "by medical men very much like other diseases . . . Medical men regard [mental illness] only in its physical aspect, they consider their duty finished when they exhaust the kind of medication supposed to be most efficacious for the purpose . . . something more is necessary to insure the highest success even to the medical treatment" (Ray 1863, p. 317). What was proposed instead was

> a system, at once gentle, philosophical, and practical, to meliorete the conditions of the insane. The primary object is to treat the patients so far as their condition will possibly admit as if they were still in the enjoyment of the healthy exercise of their mental faculties. An important desideratum for the attainment of this object is to make their conditions as boarders as comfortable as possible; that they may be the less sensible of the deprivations to which they are subjected via removed from home. Nor is it less essential to extend them the privilege or the right of as much liberty, as much freedom from personal restraint as is compatible with their safety, the safety of others, and the judicious frustrations of other branches of gerative treatment. The courtesies of civilized and social life are not to be forgotten extending as they do to the promotion of the first great object already mentioned, and operating to no inconsiderable extent, as a mean of effecting restoration to mental health. [Earle 1848, p. 26]

Moral treatment stressed that the goal of treatment is to encourage and facilitate the use by the patient of his remaining healthy faculties. The "insanity" was taken for granted, and focus of the patient's experience in the moral treatment centers was on education, manual labor, and physical exercise. Often repeated was the belief that the illness is intimately bound to the personal life of the patient; although it perhaps could not be cured, the moral treatment could allow the person to live a useful life. It was said of Dr. Butler, an early advocate of moral treatment: "It was his common practice to dig deeply into the family and personal history of his patients to establish if possible a connection between their mental disorder and some accident or err in their lives. And this he did not only that he might more intelligently treat the patient but that he might be able to give the patient and friends in case of recovery such warnings of subsequent attacks might be prevented or at least guarded against" (Page 1900, p. 49). The actual day to day inpatient care of the insane reflected this attitude of respect and tolerance for the illness: "[Dr. Butler] did not depend upon restraint or seclusion to arrest destructive habits. If a woman tore her dress he aimed to stimulate her self-respect and pride. He would provide her with a new dress conspicuous for its pretty pattern or bright colors. And when he saw her thus clad, he would express pride and pleasure, complimenting her on her improved appearance" (Page 1900, pp. 481–482). Firmness with kindness was perhaps the persistent motto of moral psychiatry. As Isaac Ray explained:

> The peculiar restlessness of the insane which impels them to roam about regardless of time and occasion, at the risk of their own safety and the peace of society, and which finds no sufficient restriction in the arrangements of an ordinary dwelling short of confinement in a small apartment, is effectually controlled in a hospital; while the range of ample galleries and airing-courts prevents that control from being oppressive and unhealthy. Their fitful humors, their wild caprices, their impulsive movements, their angry looks, are met by the steady and straightforward will of attendants who have learned to perform their duty unbiased by fear or favor. Having no object of their own to serve; imbibing the spirit of kindness which prevails around them; deterred from improper practices by a vigilant supervision, and aided by suitable architectural contrivances, they are enabled to manage their charge with the least possible degree of annoyance. Thus withdrawn from outward excitements, and especially from the persons and scenes connected with his mental disorder, the patient naturally becomes calmer, his mind opens to better suggestions, and finally seeks for repose in amusement or labor. And thus it happens that in many cases but little more is necessary to conduct the morbid process to a successful issue, besides giving the constitution a fair chance to exert its restorative powers, unembarrassed by adverse influences. [1863, pp. 321–322]

The success of moral psychiatry was impressive even by modern standards. A study of the annual reports of the Worcester Hospital in Massachusetts by Bockoven (1972) reveals that during the period 1833–1852, 1,618 of 2,267 patients whose illness had lasted less than one year prior to admission were discharged as recovered or improved (sixty-six percent recovered, five percent improved). For all patients, including those admitted with an illness lasting more than one year, fifty-nine percent were discharged as recovered or improved during this same period.

Medical or Scientific Psychiatry

The disappearance of moral treatment and the onset of "scientific" psychiatry in the late nineteenth century are said to have been due to several causes. The death of many of the charismatic founders of the moral treatment movement in the middle of the nineteenth century left the movement without eloquent spokesmen. Unfortunately, the training and education of young psychiatrists was never well formalized, and few were available to replace the early leaders. More importantly, the late nineteenth century saw an extraordinary influx of immigrants to the eastern states of America, greatly overtaxing and overburdening the existing psychiatric facilities. Terms such as "foreign insane pauperism" became established psychiatric diagnoses in annual reports. And in hospitals the kind, attentive care of earlier years gave way to woefully inadequate attempts to cope with the burgeoning population of the institutions.

Concomitant with these developments was the rising influence of scientific medicine:

> Advocates of moral treatment have very diligently inculcated the idea that they alone, by education, by experience, and by general aptitude are qualified to take the medical superintendence of the unfortunate class of patients in question and that restraint and separation from friends and acquaintances are measures in themselves which are specially curative in their influence. It will be among the chief objects of this memoir to show that these are erroneous; that the medical profession [outside the hospital] is a body fully as capable of treating cases of insanity as cases of any other disease and that in many instances sequestration is not only unnecessary but positively injurious. [Hammond 1879, quoted in Bockoven, p. 29]

John Grey, the editor of the *American Journal of Insanity* and superintendent of the Utica Hospital for over thirty years, was a prime example of this new breed of psychiatrist. He argued in his writings that insanity was due to a physical lesion, and he was a vigorous advocate of such scientific advances as introducing the microscope into American mental hospitals. Dr. Grey acquired international fame in the trial of Guideau, President Garfield's assassin, for testifying that crime and depravity were not insanity and for thus helping to convict Guideau of the assassination.

But perhaps the most important figure in the establishment of the scientific method in psychiatry was Emil Kraepelin. Kraepelin brought organization and conceptual clarity out of what previously had been much diagnostic disarray and confusion. He postulated "dementia praecox" as a medical illness and attempted to identify a characteristic onset, clinical course, and inevitable outcomes. Further, he assumed that as a medical illness it must have an organic etiology. "Obvious as may be the clinical resemblance of this disease to general paralysis in many respects, it has proved impossible so far to discover any external injurious influence which may have produced it. We only know that the years of physical development formed a favorable soil in which the disease may break out, as is also the case in maniacal-depressive insanity. The absence of external causes in this disease . . . might perhaps suggest that we have an illness in which the final cause must be sought in the metabolism disturbances of the tissue" (1904).

Kraepelin's medical-scientific approach as it has come down to us focuses on accurate clinical description, including chemical and physiologic laboratory studies if available, delineation of a specific illness state that is derived from an equally specific etiologic cause, and prediction of the course of the illness and its eventual outcome. The presumed etiology for those who use this approach is usually organic, and a specific treatment is sought, one intended to cure the specific etiogenic factor. Some have questioned the Kraepelinian assumption that an organic hypothesis of insanity is the only possible outcome of the application of the scientific method—a doubt which I share. Nonetheless, the Kraepelinian approach as it has been applied in psychiatry has generally had an exclusively organic orientation.

Personality Analysis

The approach that I shall call personality analysis can be traced back at least to Adolf Meyer's "psychobiology," which strongly influenced American psychiatry to broaden its view of mental illness. Most important, however, was Harry Stack Sullivan, who demonstrated through many years of careful work with very ill patients that psychotic persons could indeed benefit from intensive psychotherapy:

> [As soon as the acute systems have subsided] the therapist should work on *reconstructing the actual chronology of the psychosis*. All tendencies to "smooth over" the events are discouraged, and free associational techniques are introduced at intervals to fill in "failures of memories". The role of significant persons and their doings is emphasized, the patient being constantly under the influence of the formulation above set forth—*viz.*, that however mysteriously the phenomenon originated, everything that has befallen him is related to his actual living among the relatively small number of significant people, and a relatively simple course of events. Psychotic phenomena recalled from the more disturbed period are subjected to study as to their relation to these people. Dreams are studied under this guide. During this phase of the work, the patient may or may not grasp the dynamics . . . One of perhaps three situations now develops. Firstly, if the patient is doing very well, the family insists on taking him home, and generally ignores advice as to further treatment. Secondly, the chronology of the course of recent events running into psychosis is rather well recovered, and the patient is found to have great difficulty in coming to insight. He is then discharged in the regular treatment at the hands of a suitable psychoanalyst, experienced in the psychiatry of schizophrenia—and not too rigid in devotion to technique. Thirdly . . . [there is] so much growth of insight that sessions are shifted gradually to a close approximation to regular analytic sessions that follow a liberal variant of the orthodox technique. [1962, pp. 287–288]

In the 1940s and 50s, several psychoanalytically-oriented hospitals, perhaps the most famous being Chestnut Lodge in Maryland, courageously pursued intensive psychotherapeutic treatment. Therapists such as Freida Fromm-Reichman (1950) and later Harold Searles (1965) write of their attempts to reconstruct the complex and disordered internal worlds of psychotic patients. The most elegant recent statement of this approach is

Schizophrenia and the Need–Fear Dilemma (1969) by Burnham, Gladstone, and Gibson, which describes their psychotherapeutic work with severely ill patients at Chestnut Lodge.

Personality analysis applies the insights of psychodynamic and psychoanalytic thinking to the psychotic experience. It focuses on the patient as being a product of disordered and abnormal developmental experiences, and it relies heavily on intensive psychotherapy to understand these processes. Personality analysis has also strongly introduced the ethic that the hospitalization is only the initial stage in what is hoped to be a long-term psychotherapeutic effort.

Milieu Therapy

Unquestionably, one of the most influential recent treatment developments has been the concept of the "therapeutic community" or "milieu treatment." After World War II numerous investigators such as Stanton and Schwartz (1954) and Caudhill (1958) became interested in studying psychiatric wards as social systems, but the most important clinical description was that of Maxwell Jones in England. In *The Therapeutic Community* (1953) Jones describes the establishment of an open hospital ward in which the primary focus was on group interaction rather than on somatic therapy or individual psychotherapy. Jones stressed the social and interpersonal nature of each patient's impairment and the necessity for tailoring the inpatient experience toward alteration of social behaviors. To this end he used innovations such as daily community meetings, group decision making, and "reeducation" lectures on psychological topics. Jones treated primarily military veterans with "effort syndrome"—men who had received psychiatric discharges from the British military forces. In our current terminology, most of his patients appear from his description to have various character and situational disorders, and very few seem to have had a psychotic level of pathology.

What is most striking today about Jones's efforts at community resocialization is the mobilization of intense group pressure upon the patients: "The more the patient culture approximates to the unit culture, as represented by the staff, the greater will be our effectiveness in treating patients." Perhaps in the 1970s we are less certain of the unquestioned value and veracity of our own staff culture than were Jones and his colleagues in the 1940s. In any case, Jones clearly demonstrated the extraordinary power of group pressure within a psychiatric unit to change the behavior of residents toward what was felt to be more desirable by the staff.

The idea of the therapeutic community has greatly influenced inpatient treatment in this country. There are very few inpatient wards of any type that do not in some way describe themselves as a therapeutic community or therapeutic milieu. The militancy with which the ideology of therapeutic communities has been propounded can be seen in some of the more exhortative and inspirational literature of that persuasion—for example, Margolis' book, *Patient Power* (1973). On the other hand, there have been at least a few more sophisticated attempts to understand the role of community and social interaction in residential treatment centers, such as the writings of Moos (1974), Almond (1974), and Dimsdale (1975). The concept of a therapeutic community clearly grows out of the notion that all behavior—including such psychopathological behavior as schizophrenia—grows out of interpersonal transactions and that all meaningful treatment must take place in a social context.

The Existential View

Existentialism, a major branch of philosophy throughout this century, has influenced thinking in psychiatry no less than in numerous other fields. Evolving largely out of the phenomenologic school, existentialism found its first important voice in psychiatry through the clear and detailed presentation of psychopathology by Karl Jaspers. Psychiatrists such as Binswanger and Minkowski (May 1958) further explored the notion that within the mental illness experience itself lay the path of understanding. Emotional illness, the existentialists argued, could only be understood as a unique human experience, not "labeled" or "classified" as the scientific tradition in psychiatry has tended to do. Instead, existentialism has emphasized an ontological viewpoint, that is, it has attempted to understand "being" itself, rather than what are seen as artificially constructed "essences"—such as "signs," "symptoms," or "typical characteristics." Existentialists attempt to deal with human beings not as objects but as actively experiencing fellow subjects. Insofar as we observe, classify, attach labels, or categorize, we are objectifying and dehumanizing other persons. An existential critique of scientific psychiatry would stress the importance of the "I," the actively experiencing self with its own intentionality and autonomy, and would suggest that too often a scientific approach to psychopathology sees this self as a passive victim of biological or psychological processes.

The existential approach attempts empathically to understand subjective human experience, including the psychopathologic experience. The experience of insanity grows out of the individual's "life-historical process" and can only be understood in this way. If therapists listen to their patients without a scientific bias, they hear the humanness of the patients come alive, and only then can they be therapeutic in the truest sense of the word.

> Existential analysis treats the patient's utterances quite seriously and with no more prejudice or bias than in ordinary conversation with normal people . . . Existential analysis refused absolutely to examine pathological expressions with a view to seeing whether they are bizarre, absurd, illogical, or otherwise defective; rather it attempts to understand the particular world of experience to which these experiences point and how this world is formed and how it falls apart . . . The existential analyst refrains from evaluation of any kind . . . From the careful and tireless experience of what is an entirely empirical way—the patient's transformed and different ways of existence becomes clear . . . From a description given by the patients themselves regarding the changes in their world of experience, their various expressions, hallucinations, gestures, and movements can be logically understood in detail. [M. Bleuler, quoted in May 1958, p. 124]

Current Conceptual Derivatives

Out of the five clinical traditions that I have alluded to have arisen the current range of approaches to schizophrenia, which will be presented briefly here and in much more detail throughout this volume.

Moral Treatment and the Rehabilitation Approach
The rehabilitative aspect of treating persons with schizophrenia is, it seems to me, closely akin to the moral tradition of psychiatry. Despite the tremendous strides that have been made in recent years in our knowledge of schizophrenia, few people would disagree with the statement that we are as yet far from having the ability to cure this disease. A large part of our task as clinicians is still essentially to attempt rehabilitation.

Rehabilitation is based on the assumption that one is in the presence of a permanent impairment of functioning, and seeks to nurture and develop those strengths that remain relatively intact despite the impairment. In particular, the rehabilitative approach attempts to deal with those secondary areas of impairment which, rather than deriving from the primary pathology, are rather sequelae of the hypothetical primary pathologic process. For example, a secondary dysfunction in schizophrenia might be loss of a job and the necessity for vocational rehabilitation—moral psychiatry is, after all, the source of all those basket-weaving jokes. Of course, an important clinical point lies beneath the basket-weaving orientation in moral psychiatry: what a patient *does*—working in the occupational therapy shop, going with a group on an activity off the ward, helping to prepare a meal—often has a far more important impact on the patient than anything else that happens on the ward.

Teaching this rehabilitative view to psychiatric residents is not always easy. I can recall my own disappointment as a first year resident when the focus of treatment for a schizophrenic patient seemed to imply severely limiting the horizons of my therapeutic zeal and aiming for only very modest goals and accomplishments for the patient. Perhaps there is a certain curative fantasy that drives future physicians into medical school, and our hopes of "curing" patients are not easily given up. In any event, occupational therapists and social workers, either by inclination or training, seem much more comfortable with a rehabilitative orientation than do physicians—and frequently play a more important role than we do in the improvement of the most severely impaired schizophrenic patients.

What I wish to stress is that rehabilitation plays a major part in our treatment of schizophrenic patients today, just as it did when it alone was effectively used by the moral psychiatrists. My definition of the term "rehabilitation" is very similar to Siegler and Osmond's "impaired model" of treatment (1974). Tucker and Maxmen (1973), in an excellent article several years ago in the *American Journal of Psychiatry*, also stressed the rehabilitative function of inpatient wards. In this book Dr. Borus will have the most to say about rehabilitative approaches as he discusses the issues of schizophrenia and the community. Indeed, as Bockoven (1972) has suggested, it is community psychiatry that is perhaps the true heir to the moral tradition.

Medical-Scientific Approach

The medical-scientific approach views schizophrenia as a specific toxic disease arising out of a hypothetical single (or perhaps multiple) etiologic source. In this view the origins of schizophrenia ought to be essentially independent of personality, family structure, socioeconomic level, and all other similar background noise. In each of their chapters, Drs. Kety, Creese, and Hollister review in detail some new, impressive advances in the genetics, biochemistry, and pharmacotherapy of schizophrenia. This progress gives us hope that some day a specific neurochemical abnormality may be identified in schizophrenia that will allow us to prevent its occurence or at least to palliate its effects much better than we are currrently able to do.

On the other hand, an overdependence on the medical-scientific approach to schizophrenia may be severely limiting at the present time. Despite the fact that there are virtual libraries full of research on the organic basis of schizophrenia, we still have little notion of its organic etiology; prognostic indicators, though having some statistical validity in large patient populations, are all too often incorrect for individual patients; and at best biological modalities are palliative rather than curative. The point I wish to make is that while the medical-scientific approach has an important place in our understanding of schizophrenia, the actual treatment of a person with schizophrenia must consist of a wide range of personal and social interventions.

Personality Analysis

What I wish to call personality analysis is the specific psychotherapeutic technique that sees personality structure, with all its developmental antecedents, as intimately linked to schizophrenic symptoms. It is important to distinguish this type of psychotherapy from other psychotherapeutic approaches, for example, from the forms of psychotherapy practiced in rehabilitative work with patients or in strictly pharmacologic treatment. In both these approaches the clinician talks with patients no less than does the clinician in more traditional psychotherapy, and perhaps just as regularly. What is distinct to personality treatment is that the psychotherapist talks with the patient with the specific goal of coming to share with the patient some understanding of the mental contents—conscious or, depending on the orientation of the therapist, sometimes unconscious—which currently and developmentally make up the schizophrenic syndrome. Further, it is hoped that this particular psychotherapeutic process might help palliate the disorder.

Careful, dedicated therapists such as Peter Giovacchini (1967) and Harold Searles (1965) in America and much of the British school of Kleinian thinking (Segal 1964) and object relations (Guntrip 1968) feel strongly that extended psychotherapy can effect significant improvement in schizophrenia. Dr. Lidz reviews in chapter 4 some of the theoretical background of such work. Dr. Schwartz in chapter 9 writes movingly about this sort of careful, sensitive, and often frustrating and lengthy psychotherapy with psychotic patients. Many clinicians have similar experiential data from their own practices; yet the evidence from controlled studies remains conflicting as to precisely where and how personality-oriented psychotherapy can play a role in the treatment of schizophrenia. Until such evidence does exist, clinicians are forced to rely on their intuition about which schizophrenic patients have the "psychological mindedness" to benefit from such psychotherapeutic work.

Milieu Therapy

Milieu therapy has come to have a multitude of meanings. At one extreme there exists classical therapeutic communities that very closely follow Maxwell Jones's original description and often take a militant ideological stance in favor of complete group decision making in every aspect of treatment. At the other side of the spectrum are the more rational wards, perhaps better labeled "therapeutic environments," where certain milieu modalities are selectively utilized. The common denominator of all milieu orientations is a belief in the positive therapeutic benefits of social interaction. The hope is that positive social experiences during an inpatient stay will translate into improved social functioning outside the ward. As a recent excellent review by Van Putten (1976) demonstrates, however, the evidence for such effectiveness is meager. Clearly, whenever therapeutic milieus have replaced custodial wards, clinical improvement has taken place in significant numbers of schizophrenic patients. On the other hand, not only is there little evidence that milieu therapy in itself is superior to other forms of treatment such as drugs or psychotherapy, but there is also increasing concern among clinicians (such as myself) about undesirable side effects of this method of therapy (Shershow 1977b). One of these side effects is the development of group dependence; many patients, especially schizophrenic patients, may regress to a dependence on the milieu itself rather than learn to deal effectively with the outside world—a phenomenon Dr. Sonn and I call the immersion experience. The other side effect is an increase in psychotic manifestations as a result of the overstimulation of milieu treatment on the more aggressive wards; the constant series of group meetings, confrontations, and interpretations may actually be harmful for schizophrenic patients. Although the mobilization of peer pressure may be a powerful and effective modality for other sorts of patients—witness its relative effectiveness among communities of drug addicts—with schizophrenia the inpatient milieu must, in my opinion, be much more individualized.

Existential Treatment
Finally, existentialism helps us confront honestly the reality of the schizophrenia experience in the persons that we face in clinical practice. In recent years perhaps the best known writings that utilize existential concepts to understand psychotic phenomena are those of R. D. Laing (1960) and Rollo May (1958). Loren Mosher in chapter 10 writes about the Soteria residential treatment community for schizophrenia in San Francisco, where schizophrenic patients are allowed to live through the acute psychotic phase without the intrusion of medications and with minimal social controls and limits. Such an experiment demonstrates

that despite the "abnormal" behavior and affects associated with what we call schizophrenia, there remains the possibility of an experiencing self that can be helped to survive the process without utilization of the more aggressive and intrusive therapeutic techniques that are commonplace today.

For me, the existential concept is a healthy antidote to what seems an inevitable clinical impulse to objectify patients. Such objectification, existentialism continually reminds us, may contain elements of dehumanization. We may, if we wish, view our patients as "sick," but they are also fellow human beings undergoing a strange and frightening experience—and an experience that *may* be growth producing. Insofar as we fail to consider this possibility, and exclusively see the schizophrenic process as destructive, we fail to respond empathically to the basically human process we are observing.

It seems to me that the crucial question for clinicians at this time is whether or not we can sustain the variety of approaches I have outlined. Historical parallels are always hazardous; yet it is hard not to see similarities between our time and a century ago, when the scientific revolution overthrew moral psychiatry. Will we repeat the unfortunate and sadly ironic consequences that grew out of abandoning the profoundly personal and humane methods of moral psychiatry? In my view, the broadly catholic stance that has characterized American psychiatry during the past several decades is jeopardized most of all by a current tendency among some to abdicate this pluralism.

For indeed, these diverse conceptions *do* make significant and practical differences in the treatment of any patient, but particularly schizophrenic patients. Further, our conceptions will become important on a larger scale as third party insurers and government financing of health care increasingly determine the quality and nature of the resources used for the care of schizophrenia. Is schizophrenia a toxic illness or a way of life? To what extent do the symptoms of schizophrenia relate to preexisting personality and development? Does intervention on a social or economic level have a significant impact on the disease process? These are but a few of the questions whose explicit (or implicit) answers will enormously influence future treatment.

In this volume one will find, then, not unity or synthesis but stark disagreements, reflecting the widely varying conceptual stances that each investigator or clinician brings to bear on schizophrenia. If any comfort is to be had in such diversity of approach, as Dr. Savodnik points out in chapter 2, it may only be in the knowledge that much of the diversity reflects basic intellectual rifts in western culture and in its philosophy of science.

As clinicians we can only attempt to participate in the variety of approaches, even if such a task often seems to strain the limits of the most flexible among us. We are both scientists and humane practitioners; it is hoped that the essays herein will be of some assistance in bearing this double burden.

REFERENCES

Almond, R. 1974. *The healing community*. New York: Jason Aronson.

Bleuler, E. 1924. *Textbook of psychiatry*. Trans. A. A. Brill. New York: Macmillan.

Bockoven, J. S. 1972. *Moral treatment in community mental health*. New York: Springer.

Burnham, D., A. Gladstone, and R. Gibson. 1969. *Schizophrenia and the need—fear dilemma*. New York: International Universities Press.

Caudhill, W. 1958. *The psychiatric hospital as a small society*. Cambridge: Harvard University Press.

Dimsdale, J. E. 1975. Goals of therapy on psychiatric impatient units. *Social Psychiatry* 10:1–7.

Earle, P. 1848. *History, description, and statistics of the Bloomingdale Asylum for the Insane*. New York: Egbert, Hovey, and King.

Fromm-Reichman, F. 1950. *Principles of intensive psychotherapy*. Chicago: University of Chicago Press.

Giovacchini, P., and B. Boyer. 1967. *Psychoanalytic treatment of characterological and schizophrenic disorders*. New York: Science House.

Guntrip, H. 1968. *Schizoid phenomenon, object relations, and the self*. New York: International Universities Press.

Jaspers, K. 1963. *General psychopathology*. Chicago: University of Chicago Press.

Jones, M. 1953. *The therapeutic community*. New York: Basic Books.

Kernberg, O. 1975. *Borderline conditions and pathological narcissism*. New York: Jason Aronson.

Kohut, H. 1974. *The analysis of the self*. New York: International Universities Press.

Kraepelin, E. 1904. *Lectures on clinical psychiatry*. London: Baillière, Tindall, and Cox.

Laing, R. D. 1960. *The divided self*. Chicago: Quadrangle Books.

Margolis, P. 1973. *Patient power*. Springfield: Charles C. Thomas.

May, R., E. Angel, and H. Ellenberger. 1958. *Existence*. New York: Simon and Schuster.

Meyer, A. 1950. *The collected papers*. Baltimore: Johns Hopkins University Press.

Moos, R. H. 1974. *Evaluating treatment environments*. New York: Wiley Interscience.

Page, C. 1901. John Butler: the man and his hospital methods. *American Journal of Insanity* 52:477–492.

Ray, I. 1863. *Mental Hygiene*. Boston: Ticknor and Fields.

Searles, H. 1965. *Collected papers on schizophrenia*. New York: International Universities Press.

Segal, H. 1964. *An introduction to the works of Melanie Klein*. New York: Basic Books.

Siegler, M., and H. Osmond. 1974. *Models of madness, models of medicine*. New York: Macmillan.

Shershow, J. C. 1977a. *Delicate branch: the vision of moral psychiatry*. New York: Dabor Science Publishing.

_____. 1977b. Disestablishing a therapeutic community. *Current Concepts in Psyciatry* 3:8–11.

Sonn, M., and J. C. Shershow. Unpublished. Immersion and distance: two varieties of experience of psychiatric hospitalization.

Stanton, A., and M. Schwartz. 1954. *The mental hospital*. New York: Basic Books.

Sullivan, H. S. 1962. *Schizophrenia as a human process*. New York: Norton.

Tucker, G. J., and J. S. Maxmen. 1973. The practice of hospital psychiatry: a formulation. *American Journal of Psychiatry* 130:887–891.

Van Putten, T. 1976. Milieu treatment of the schizophrenias. In *Treatment of schizophrenia: progress and prospects*, ed. L. G. West and D. E. Flinn. New York: Grune and Stratton.

2

The Manifest and the Scientific Images

IRWIN SAVODNIK

On the subject of schizophrenia, the problem child of psychiatry, disagreement serves as a euphemistic guise for unlimited confusion. This confusion is not restricted to such substantive issues as etiology, pathogenesis, and the like, but also extends to the very methodological and conceptual schemes used to organize what we take to be knowledge about the subject. And this lack of unanimity about the manner in which the so-called facts of schizophrenia are arranged leads to considerable controversy about the methods whereby the phenomena related to schizophrenia are investigated. Furthermore, psychiatrists themselves are often at a loss to clarify how issues are conceptually related and what distinguishes them methodologically and theoretically.

It seems to me that all the major issues confronting psychiatry as a discipline within contemporary medicine converge on the problem of schizophrenia, and as a result our resources are strained to the limit when we attempt to provide a coherent picture of the phenomena that fall under the denotation of that term.* How should psychiatrists conceive of their enterprise

* This conflict bears similarities to the controversy that surrounded various attempts to explain the phenomena included in the concept of aphasia. Because aphasia could not be readily conceptualized by the available theories of neural organization, it was necessary to construct a more sophisticated view of the central nervous system. In particular, the notion of strictly localizable areas of the brain that subserved functions related to speech, reading, writing, computation, spatial imagery, and active thought, while adequate for explaining various other phenomena, was shown to be grossly inadequate in accounting for aphasia. This

and, concomitantly, how ought they to conceive of themselves as members in this noble effort? Answers to these questions pose a serious problem, indeed perhaps the ultimate problem, for the psychiatrist, because they question the very existence of psychiatry as a discipline with its own conceptual foundations. If psychiatry is to be more than the application of the principles of medicine, neurology, and so forth, and more than a sophisticated psychology, then just what it is to be is illuminated by the problem of schizophrenia.

A current controversy within psychiatry exemplifies the conceptual confusion that is dominating the field. The two contrasting positions are known by a variety of terms; I will refer to them as objective-descriptive psychiatry and, for lack of a better term, dynamic psychiatry.

Objective-Descriptive Psychiatry

This position is derived from the work of Emil Kraepelin, a German psychiatrist of the late nineteenth and early twentieth centuries who developed an approach to psychiatric disorders that is regarded as the foundation stone of the medical model in contemporary psychiatry (Kraepelin 1915; 1968; Havens 1973). The Kraepelinians, or more specifically the neo-Kraepelinians (Woodruff 1974), assert that schizophrenia is a disease like any other disease, having an etiology, pathogenesis, course, prognosis, and outcome. In making this assertion the neo-Kraepelinians move the study of schizophrenia directly into the mainstream of medicine. Schizophrenia might be, as some have called it, a problem in living, but to the objective-descriptive school of psychiatry it is a problem in living much like congestive heart failure or pyelonephritis. According to this model, the schizo-

---

model of the brain was replaced by a more sophisticated relational model based on the concept of the reflex organization of the central nervous system. Still later, the holistic model was put forth. These increasingly sophisticated models of neural function are a testimony to the need for more subtle considerations in the face of a central clinical and theoretical problem. Similarly, in the case of schizophrenia, simple solutions analogous to the strict localization model or the reflex model are not satisfying and may not be adequate for the tasks that psychiatry sets for itself. (See Bastian 1898; Goldstein 1948; Jackson 1958; Lucia 1970; Geschwind 1965a; 1965b.)

phrenic is sick. He *has* a disease and, as in the study of all other diseases, the physician ought to look for the objective signs that point to the existence of the disorder. If this disease is mythical as some would have it, then so is arteriosclerosis, infectious hepatitis, and carcinoma of the lung. Furthermore, the etiology of schizophrenia is thought to be organic. Whether this latter point is essential to the Kraepelinian position or only accidental is problematic, but certainly the current population of neo-Kraepelinian psychiatrists are largely in favor of an organic explanation for the occurrence of schizophrenic behavior. And in the spirit of Kraepelin himself, neo-Kraepelinian psychiatry is highly taken, if not obsessed, with the task and problem of classifying schizophrenic behavior.

Some insight into the neo-Kraepelinian mode of thinking may be gained by seeing what it is *not* concerned with. I would like to mention three broad areas of nonconcern. In the first place, the neo-Kraepelinian psychiatrist is not terribly interested in the problem of character insofar as that term in understood from, say, the novels of Henry James or Dostoyevsky. What interest there seems to be in character revolves around specific disorders of personality and is discussed strictly in terms of the observable constituents of the disorder. As far as a theory of character goes, there is none.* Presumably, there is some faith in the hypothesis that various characterological differences result from differences of neurological organization that are secondary to genetic differences (Slater and Cowie 1971; Hook 1973). The nonconcern with character lies, I think, in the fact that the term itself is highly psychological in that it does not lend itself very readily to a neurological or biochemical reduction or transformation. Since neo-Kraepelinians regard themselves as "hard scientists," the embracing of categories whose "scientific" legitimacy is problematic is itself a dubious action. Character, then, is of interest only to the extent that we can speak of the objectively identifiable constituents of it and no more. Insofar as character might be regarded in a broad sense as a moral posture in the world, as the

---

* For instance, in Woodruff's book (1974) the index makes no reference to character. Personality is dealt with only through a discussion of "the anti-social personality." No general or theoretical point of view is offered other than the overall medical approach to the phenomenon.

capacity to do otherwise, or as a life script determined by past individual experience, the objective-descriptive psychiatrist has little if anything to say.

The second general area of nonconcern for the neo-Kraepelinian is human intention. Intention really has two important senses. One is derived from the psychology of Brentano (1874), who thought that every mental act involves a distinction between an act and an object, so that thinking is not *merely* thinking, but thinking *of* some entity, idea, or whatever. Included in this sense of intention is the notion that a person has an intention to perform a certain kind of action, a mental proclivity towards a certain kind of conscious, goal-directed behavior. The intentionalist in this context argues for the irreducibility of mental concepts to material ones. That is, the psychological dimension of human existence is thought by the intentionalist to be unexpressible or not entirely expressible in terms of the material particles that constitute the physical world. (See Land 1876; Flint 1876; James 1950; Russell 1959.)

The other sense of intention refers to meaning; in broad scope it pertains to the variety of symbolic usages that constitute our various expressive modalities of thought and speech. This notion of intentionality is particularly mentalistic in that meaning itself is an inherently mentalistic term not lending itself very readily to a physicalist interpretation. (See Anscombe 1957; Harré and Secord 1973; Chisholm 1957.) The neo-Kraepelinian is not really concerned with this second sense of intentionality because it involves a strong element of personal interpretation that is not amenable to standard procedures of scientific investigation. As for the first sense of the term, the neo-Kraepelinian recognizes it only in its most narrow sense, that is, he will admit to the goal-directedness of human behavior.* But this admission is really not very committal since most scientists will admit, at one level or another to the goal-directedness of a good deal of organic behavior. Hence, the human being, as far as intentionality is con-

---

* The philosophical support for the Kraepelinian is formidable and seen in the covering law model of explanation put forth by Hempel (1942). In the same subsumption-theoretic sense, Rosenbluth, Wiener, and Bigelow (1943) propose a causalist account of purposiveness, using the cybernetic concept of negative feedback. See also Nagel (1951; 1961) and Braithwaite (1953).

cerned, is not distinguished from other species in the eyes of the objective-descriptive psychiatrist.

The third area of nonconcern has to do with individual history, in which neo-Kraepelinians have only the most stereotyped and attenuated interest. They regard the individual as a container for the disease process. Hence, the individual is of interest only with respect to the particular variations that a given disease manifests. That is, it is the host response, so to speak, that is of interest to the neo-Kraepelinian rather than the host. (By contrast, Kraepelin himself was very interested in individual history and saw the varieties of schizophrenic presentation as a function of variations in the individual lives of the people who were so afflicted.) Concepts related to the notion of individual history such as developmental stages, epigenesis, and intrapsychic conflict are, for the most part, not taken seriously by neo-Kraepelinians.

What, then, are the philosophical underpinnings upon which the neo-Kraepelian position in psychiatry rests? It is reassuring, at least at first, to point out that these psychiatrists, insofar as their philosophy is concerned, are in rather good company. Quine (1960; 1970) and to a significant extent Skinner (1972) would both have considerable sympathy with the entire neo-Kraepelinian enterprise. In addition, neo-Kraepelinians are essentially physicalists in that their antimentalistic approach to psychiatry is consonant with a good deal of contemporary anti-Cartesian philosophy. Some of the philosophical groundwork, as well as ultimate philosophical implications, might be stated in the following way: the world is essentially and entirely a material domain and all knowledge is amenable to the methods of science. As in anti-Cartesian philosophy, mental entities such as minds, ideas, meanings, and the like are not admitted into this position's ontological framework. There is only one kind of knowledge and that is the knowledge which science as we conceive it constructs. It is not a theory of logical positivism; the theory of meaning that logical positivism puts forth is rejected both because it is a theory of *meaning* and also because the verifiability principle that lies at the heart of this theory is itself not verifiable. There is no science of the mental, and the idea of psychic dynamics in a psychoanalytic sense is, for such a position, utterly unnecessary. What needs to be said about human beings can be said using the materialistic language of science and no reference to intentional or mentalistic entities needs to be made (Quine 1960; Schuldenfrei 1972).*

Finally—and this involves more of a philosophical implication than an actual state of affairs—this view of a scientific approach to man embraces the idea of an extensionalist language, that is, a language which is purely denotative, devoid of any connotative or "meaningful" references. The hallmark of such a language is what Quine calls substitutivity, and he points out some of the difficulties one runs into when one's language is intentional or meaning laden rather than extensional. As Quine would have it, purging our language of intentional content is a healthy thing insofar as our scientific enterprise is concerned. Consider, for example, the statement, "There is a pile of salt on the table." Presumably, as good empiricists we could substitute for the everyday word "salt" the term "NaCl" and restate the assertion as, "There is a pile of NaCl on the table." But we run into problems when we have a statement with a mentalistic term contained within, that is, a propositional attitude. In the case of the assertion, "I believe there is a pile of salt on the table," we cannot simply replace "salt" with "NaCl," since I may know or believe that salt is on the table but not know or believe that NaCl is on the table. Hence, from the perspective of Quinean materialism, the employment of an unambiguous, nonmentalistic vocabulary and the purging of mentalistic or psychological references in the domain of psychiatry is ultimately a healthy and growth-stimulating procedure that avoids pitfalls such as referential opacity, "vagaries of reference," and a "double standard" between intentional and extensional modes of discourse.

I would like to suggest two areas of criticism of the objective-descriptive or neo-Kraepelinian psychiatrist. We know from ex-

---

* While this is a general statement of some broad aspects of Quinean philosophy, certain aspects of this position are deliberately left vague. For instance, Quine's (1970) adoption of a Duhemian position (1962) is not addressed here and is problematic in that opponents of objective-descriptive psychiatry often appeal to a Duhemian analysis to defend their own position. Furthermore, the ultimate constituents of Quine's universe represent a difficult, if not unclear, part of his own philosophy. Ultimate implications for an enterprise such as psychiatry, then, are not dealt with here.

perience in dealing with schizophrenic patients that very often the patient, his family, his friends want to know "what happened." By "what happened" they do not mean how much dopamine was present in the basal ganglia of the patient's central nervous system. They mean, in terms of the person's life, experiences, and current environment, why did all this happen? The patient may ask, "Was I working myself too hard?" "Was I deprived as a child?" Others may ask, "Did we not provide some essential ingredient for his healthy development?" "Did I smother him too much?" And so on. In short, people want a psychological explanation. And they will not settle for anything else. They do not care that meaning can be done away with in Quinean fashion; they want to know the "meaning" of this affair which has so abruptly and catastrophically intruded upon their lives. They want to understand schizophrenia not as a molecular phenomenon but as a phenomenon in terms of which the everyday furniture of the universe is arranged. They want the tables and chairs of their experiences to be comprehensible to them in the same terms that they use to refer to these pieces in their everyday lives. They want to know about this phenomenon called schizophrenia in terms of the motives, intentions, desires, frustrations, disappointments, and attitudes of the individual involved. Furthermore, their fears, anxieties, and uncertainties will not be assuaged by a molecular or neurological explanation. Nor will statistical references help. What they want is an understanding of the individual in his concrete embodiment in the world.

Neo-Kraepelinian psychiatry is, it seems, quite unprepared to deal with this sort of request. It is committed, necessarily, to the reinterpretation and translation of such questions into the language of pathology, neurology, and biochemistry. Because characterological, intentional, and individual historical elements are downplayed in the understanding of the schizophrenic person, the capacity to answer such questions is severely limited. All neo-Kraepelinians can say is that such questions are poorly expressed and ought to be expressed in a language with which they are more comfortable. This is not altogether arrogant posture on their part. After all, there came a time in human history when scientists refused to explain various aspects of human behavior on the basis of possession, demonology, witchcraft, and so on. Nevertheless, unless one is committed to a radical redefinition of the meaning of human existence and as a consequence to a radical redefinition of humankind, such a position is very hard to defend. The reason I insist that a radical redefinition of the nature of humans is involved here is that I conceive us to be creatures who, as part of our nature, reflect *upon* our own nature; hence, an alteration in the substance or content of that reflection will, of necessity, alter the view we have of our nature (Droysen 1925).

Another area of criticism has to do with a certain naive conception of science that neo-Kraepelinian psychiatrists, but not their philosophical counterparts, seem to have. In the first place, there seems to be a belief that the only thing to which behavioral scientists ought to attend are observables—that is, entities such as behaviors, appearances, and laboratory findings. Picturing themselves as good empiricists, they regard their scientific enterprise as most pure when only observable entities are referred to and dealt with. The philosophical underpinning here is Machean (1893) and Comtean (1853). However, if we reflect for a moment on the explanatory power of scientific theories in general, we find something quite different from the neo-Kraepelinian paradigm. That is, what makes a scientific explanation compelling, cogent, and incisive is specifically its reference to unobservables —to the atoms, molecules, neutrinos, fields and forces of the world in which we live.* Such theoretical entities are not mere instruments of explanation but real phenomena that serve as the power behind the throne of scientific explanation. Neo-Kraepelinian psychiatry is guilty specifically of avoiding such theoretical speculation because it naively believes that in postulating unobservables it is being nonscientific.

A second problematic feature of the neo-Kraepelinian philosophy of science is what I consider a naive operationalism. This view rests in part on certain presuppositions derived from an inadequate empiricism to which, again, the neo-Kraepelinians take

---

* Sellars (1963) makes a related point in his discussion of behavior when he distinguishes between establishing statistical correlation of observable behavior and constructing explanations in terms of postulated entities or processes within the discipline of neurophysiology.

pride in subscribing but whose full implications they fail to see (Taylor 1964). There are several problems with operationalism that could be raised, but in this context it will suffice to point out two major ones. First, operationalism commits the neo-Kraepelinian to a nonpsychological account of psychology because, in its stringent adherence to "observables," it does not allow for mentalistic terms, for those terms that refer to psychological processes. Second, in the thesis of operationalism there is a circularity such that the so-called operational definition of a term requires for itself the use of the term it was meant to define.* These criticisms are, I think, rather severe and raise serious doubts as to the scientific status of a medical discipline with such a narrow conception of its own operation.

The last feature I will mention which limits the neo-Kraepelinian conception of science has to do with the so-called "myth of the given" (Sellars 1963). What is known as the foundationalist view holds that at the heart of all we know of the world are certain empirical contents. These are the atoms out of which all knowledge is built and which are unquestioned and uninferred. Thus, the neo-Kraepelinian is interested, on an ideal plane at least, in strictly observable behaviors that are uninterpreted or interpreted minimally. For example, a patient may be said to be acting bizarrely without any reference to the content of the bizarre behavior. Or a patient may be described as having a blunted affect with no reference made to the meaning of the affect as it relates, for example, to cognitive processes. Behaviors or affects are regarded as irreducible givens, empirical atoms that are observed and uninterpreted. They are simply gathered for statistical correlation. Now this would not be a terribly destructive or naive position except for the fact that it is, to put in bluntly, wrong. Such a brand of empiricism was put forth by the logical positivists in the 1930s and is still subscribed to by a few individuals today; but it has been shown to be essentially inadequate largely because what we regard as given is inherently and deeply theory-laden. We cannot simply list different behaviors without at the same time drawing in certain theoretical assump-

---

* It should be pointed out that Philip Frank (1957) argues against the circularity objection. See also Hempel (1966) and Bridgman's original statement (1927).

tions in order to both identify these behaviors and correlate them with other bits of data so that they make sense.

In sum, then, the neo-Kraepelinian is faced with some rather severe criticisms from two very different sources. The first comes from the everyday man, who wants an everyday explanation and will settle for nothing less. The second is from the philosophy of science, in the context of which the scientific position of the neo-Kraepelinian is incurably naive or incorrect. If neo-Kraepelinian psychiatry aspires to legitimacy and posterity, it must answer these criticisms in a way that it has not yet done.

Dynamic Psychiatry

I turn now to the second of the two positions, which, for want of a better term, I refer to as dynamic psychiatry. Briefly, this brand of psychiatry admits into its arena, its universe of discourse, mental events and those terms that refer to them. Psychoanalysts, interpersonal psychiatrists, and other psychotherapists are all part of dynamic psychiatry to a greater or lesser extent. This camp holds that the explanation of human behavior should be in psychological terms. Dynamic psychiatry attempts to characterize the current or contemporary state of affairs of an individual in terms of psychological states, intentions, motives, and the like; and, further, it attempts to explain the current state in terms of antecedent states that are themselves psychological rather than material. Hence, the level of discourse remains mentalistic and, to a considerable degree, Cartesian.

At the very foundation of dynamic psychiatry is a radical difference with neo-Kraepelinian thinking: the data that dynamic psychiatrists collect are different, both because of what they regard as data in the first place and because of the specific theory-ladenness of the material. But of equal importance is the contrast between the dynamic psychiatrist's and the objective-descriptive psychiatrist's views of humankind with respect to the concept of personal autonomy. The objective-descriptive psychiatrist holds that the human being is a physical entity completely controlled by the laws of physics and its particular extensions, namely, the laws of biology, biophysics, and the like. This position is consistent with that of hard determinism: the autonomy of human beings, when viewed under the aspect of all eternity, is for the most part illusory and not to be countenanced by a good scientist of human behavior. There is no real decision making, then, but only the appearance of deliberation (Feyerabend 1963). As a matter of ultimate fact, all there is is the interaction of material objects that determine the behaviors of organisms, some of whom we call human beings. The dynamic psychiatrist, to the contrary, holds that human beings are decision-making, autonomous agents who manifest not only behaviors but also actions that are the expression of intentions, motives, and desires. The individual is seen to possess an irreducible and irrefutable autonomy under the aspect of eternity and is not regarded as reducible merely to the motions of material bodies regardless of how ultimate they may be.

In order to get at the core of dynamic psychiatry and understand its conception of schizophrenia, it is helpful to examine certain aspects of its founding father, Sigmund Freud. A broad and complicated issue that I would like to take up here is the claim on the part of Freud and his followers that psychoanalysis constituted a scientific discipline with a coherent methodology and explanatory apparatus.*

Freud's scientific background was related to his education as a neurologist. He was a Helmholtzian determinist and a subscriber to Haeckel's law; he also felt the full impact of Darwin's theory of evolution. Furthermore, his understanding of the nervous system as a biological unit embodying multiple phylogenetic characteristics as well as a hierarchical structure contributed to his understanding of the psychic apparatus as being a genetic phenomenon with topographic and structural features (Rapaport 1960; Ellenberger 1970). That Freud believed the brain served as an organic foundation for all behavior is clear from his earliest

---

* It is striking to note, particularly in the light of what a neo-Freudian, Eric Erikson, has to say about the concept of psychological identity, that Freud was forty-four years old at the time the *Interpretation of Dreams* was published (Freud 1900). For most people, whatever radical changes take place in their lives usually occur prior to such an age. Yet in 1900 Freud was to publish a book which, in a brief time, would become world famous. That he regarded the *Interpretation of Dreams* as standing on firm neurological and scientific principles is without question. What is questionable, of course, is whether in fact his belief is ultimately justified.

writings. *The Project for a Scientific Psychology* (1897) was his definitive, albeit unsuccessful, attempt to delineate the relation between neurological and psychological functioning. After failing this, he wrote to his peripatetic friend Wilhelm Fliess in 1898: "I have no desire at all to leave the psychology hanging in the air with no organic basis. But, beyond the feeling of conviction [that there must be such a basis], I have nothing, either theoretical or therapeutic, to work on, and so I must behave as if confronted by just psychological factors only" (Freud 1960).

This attitude of Freud has actually persisted in psychoanalysis, although usually in highly disguised form, and is perhaps most strikingly seen in the enthusiastic response given to James Papez' classical paper on the limbic system in 1937.* This paper represented for the Freudians a proof of Freud's ultimate view that all of psychic life was firmly grounded in neurological events. The claim to science was not made by Freud or his followers merely on the basis of a reductive materialism but rather on the idea that there could be a science of the mental. It is not accidental that dynamic psychiatry has the name that it does. Both Freud and his disciples thought that principles of physics such as those found in classical Newtonian dynamics as well as those of thermodynamics operated in some form or other in the psychic apparatus. Hence, a science of the mental would reveal those laws that characterize all the various phenomena of mental life. However, Freudian metapsychology contains both intentional and extensional dimensions, and as a result, Freudianism (like Marxism in this regard) contains a peculiar admixture of accounts of the human condition.

In some ways dynamic psychiatry, or in a more limited sense, Freudian psychiatry, is modeled after the kind of explanations provided by physics and the hard sciences. Hempel's covering law model of explanation as originally put forth in 1942 characterizes this mode of accounting and is variously referred to as a nomological or law-like explanation. This model of explanation is present in the metapsychology of psychoanalysis but—and this is an important "but"—it is not the sole mode of explanation,

---

* Although Papez explored the anatomical units making up the limbic system, it was actually MacLean (1952) who first used the term "limbic system."

or more properly, of accounting. For as Rapaport (1960) points out, each of the five classes of propositions making up the meta-psychology of psychoanalysis—namely, the dynamic, economic, structural, genetic, and adaptive assumptions—is necessary but only the totality of the five classes is sufficient for a satisfactory account of a psychoanalytic explanation.

The other mode of accounting for human action is hermeneutics, which is derived from a type of antipositivist thinking that arose in the nineteenth century. The sources of this brand of idealism, as it was sometimes regarded, are German philosophers, historians, and social scientists, among them Max Weber (1949), H. Rickert (1926), Wilhelm Dilthey (1959), and J. G. Droysen (1925). These individuals attack the notion that there is one way to account for all the varieties of human experience. It is a reaction against what has been called the "methodological monism of positivism" (Von Wright 1971). They forge a distinction between nomothetic accounts, which search for underlying universal laws and are exemplified by explanations in the physical sciences, and ideographic accounts, which attempt a systematic and descriptive study of the individual. Out of this distinction grew a methodological difference that Droysen characterized by the two terms *explanation* and *understanding* (*Erklaren* and *Verstehen*). The method of understanding is different from the method of explanation, as is the form of their accounts. Understanding, for Dilthey, lay at the basis of the social sciences, what Dilthey called the *Geisteswissenschaften,* which is roughly translated as moral science. The *Verstehen* tradition, then, made use of the concept of intentionality as well as related notions of meaning, teleology, and values. To understand a human being from the point of view of *Verstehen* in contradistinction to *Erklaren,* it is necessary to see how each state or stage in the individual's life proceeds from the preceding stages, in accordance with a regularity that is based not on some universal law pertaining to all men but rather on a rule of development indigenous to the individual. To understand an individual, whether a great historical figure or a patient in a psychiatric hospital, the *Verstehen* demands that we understand the variety of "meanings" in the individual's life, so that we know what it is like to be that individual. Whether the underlying methodology of *Verstehen* is merely empathy or something more is not clear. Weber (1949) and others argued that it was considerably more, although critics such as Karl Popper (1962) seemed to regard it as a sort of softhearted and nonrigorous attempt to understand complex human events.

It is a peculiarity of dynamic (and Freudian) psychiatry that both types of accounting are present. This tension between scientific accounts, exemplified by the covering law model, and *Verstehen* is responsible for much of the seemingly problematic character of dynamic thinking. Because of this double standard, so to speak, the ability of dynamic psychiatry to predict the outcome of certain psychological states of affairs may be regarded as severely limited. However, prediction, which may be regarded as one side of explanation, is not always a goal of the account that dynamic psychiatry attempts to provide. In particular, the dynamic, economic, and structural points of view favor ordinary scientific explanation as the basis for their intelligibility, while the genetic and adaptive points of view favor the *Verstehen* accounts, although elements of both may be seen in each point of view.

Two Modes of Conduct

What, then, do we make of dynamic psychiatry and the account of human beings it provides? What critical comments might be made? I have just one. It is that all of dynamic psychiatry is very likely wrong. But being wrong must not be equated with being bad; further, there is a sense in which this point of view is wrong which gives it its value with respect to understanding the depth of human experience. However before I indicate the wrongness of this point of view and then proceed to the marriage of the two perspectives, I would like to discuss an aspect of psychiatry that probably fits best into what might be called the sociology of knowledge.

The psychiatrist is in an epistemological position that is relativized by his relation to two different kinds of people; that is, the way in which he knows or understands the subject matter of his discipline is conditioned by the people to whom he must communicate what he knows. These two groups of people are, broadly speaking, other physicians and the rest of humanity.

When the psychiatrist speaks or communicates with other doctors, by virtue of the fact that he considers himself to be part of the medical community and shares a broad scientific world view with them, he becomes "more scientific." He tends to use the language of medicine in order to explain the phenomena with which he is confronted. He will speak of catecholamines, "soft neurological signs," psychophysiological concomitants of anxiety, and the like. In short, his neo-Kraepelinian bent is exercised because he feels that the physician to whom he is speaking will regard him with the most legitimacy when this set of locutions is employed. And there is some utility in a medical terminology that is based on a broad notion of the extensional use of language. Phenomena are rendered in medical jargon because it is believed that this is the best way to present them objectively, measurably, and with the least degree of distortion. The price that is paid, however, is the loss of the language in which the experience is ordinarily described.

When the psychiatrist is confronted with the task of communicating with the rest of humanity, his language is of necessity quite different. In the first place, the rest of humanity is not assumed to be familiar with the highly technical language of medicine, neurology, and psychiatry. More important is the fact that the rest of humanity, for the most part, is not interested in hearing the catastrophes of psychiatry described in terms of humors, neurons, molecules, or whatever. Instead, people demand to be spoken to and of in people-terms. This is true not just in the case of communicating with relatives but in the process of doing what is broadly termed psychotherapy. If the psychiatrist is to communicate with the broad mass of humanity with whom he interacts as a result of his dealings with psychiatric patients, then he must be able to understand the "phenomenology" of psychiatric problems in language that is readily accessible both to himself and to other people. Such a language is, as we have seen, intentional and less than scientific. Although a certain scientific price might be paid, there is little doubt that the personal and human depth of the experience must be rendered in the terms to which our language is aptly suited.

The psychiatrist, then, be he a neo-Kraepelinian or a dynamically-oriented practitioner, is in a very difficult situation. In fact, it is this difficult situation that points up the identity crisis of psychiatry, and it is in the case of schizophrenia that emotions and issues are heightened to a maximal extent so that this identity crisis stands out most sharply. How shall the psychiatrist speak? In more mentalistic terms, how shall he think? Ought he to adopt the highly scientific and perhaps behavioral language of the neo-Kraepelinian? Or should he adopt the posture of the dynamic psychiatrist, who uses a language more closely affiliated with the phenomenology of psychiatric experiences? But it is precisely at this point that we must stop and ask ourselves a preliminary question: Is the very question itself appropriate? Or does it not, in a sense, prejudice us to think in a manner that obscures the deeper solution to this dilemma? It is my feeling that an either/or question of the sort I have just asked not only obscures the solution but actually creates the dilemma. There is simply no need for an either/or; there is, rather, a requirement that the two views be wedded to one another along the lines of a conceptual framework that is neither naive nor false.

Let us return now to the point that I raised concerning dynamic psychiatry and my assertion that it was ultimately wrong. What I meant by that was what the physicist Sir Arthur Eddington meant when he said that the table before me is really much more space than matter and what I see before me is really something of an illusion and its concomitant account is nothing more than a myth (Eddington 1949; Stebbing 1937). There is no real substantial table but rather a series of electrical particles that are in constant motion and whose interactions provide us with the experience of a substantial object before our eyes. The fact is, then, that there is no table before us but merely the illusion of one, and what really is before us, what really is the truth of the matter, is a highly complex set of molecular phenomena. The most radical of physicists will say, then, let us dispense with tables, chairs, and the literal and metaphorical furniture of our universe and learn to speak in a language that more accurately depicts the world as it really is. The problem with this radical approach, however, is a certain recalcitrance about the way in which we account for our own experiences. There is a seeming irreducibility about the furniture of our world that will not yield to such considerations, be they empirical or logical. We insist

that there are tables, chairs, and the like and will accept no substitute. Not only do we have what seems to be a psychological
need for these entities, but if we look at the problem somewhat
closer we recognize that it is the myth of the table, the myth of
the chair, the myth of the substantive object that gives the scientific image its value, its meaning, and its cogency. It is because
our everyday world is shown ultimately to be drawn along different lines that the patterns of reality falling within these lines
have any import for us at all. In a certain sense, then, perhaps not
a mere psychological sense, what seems to be the ultimate constituents of reality, be they molecules, quarks, or whatever, are
derivative in the sense that they would have little or no meaning
for us were we not to first hold on to the mythical image that we
have on an everyday level. If we return, then, to the two accounts of human beings discussed above, the same relation can
be seen between them. Let us grant the neo-Kraepelinian all that
he wants; let us say that in an ultimate sense there are neurological, indeed, molecular foundations for our acting the way we do.
But there is still the acting the way we do that must be depicted
in its own terms. If we neglect this dimension, then whatever the
Kraepelinian offers us in the way of an account is rendered
meaningless and empty. The intentional accounts of the experiences we have are the tables and chairs of our psychological universe, while the molecules, neurons, and biogenic amines are
the ultimate constituents of the world beyond the realm of appearance.

In the same sense that we cannot dispense with the ordinary
furnishings of our world in favor of a strictly ultimate or reduc-
tionist view, so we cannot dispense with the refined psychological account we have of human beings in favor of some ultimate
medical or neurological ontology. To do so would do violence to
that very ontology that we esteem so highly. At the same time,
the medical and neurological accounts add depth and dimen-
sionality to our psychological ones. It is, therefore, through a
wedding of the two positions that the deepest and most significant vision of man can be had because it is through this sort of
merger that the relevance of each account to our experiences can
be seen most clearly. With respect to schizophrenia, such a conceptual amalgamation is necessary to accommodate the diverse

patterns of phenomena and conceptual schemes that seem applicable. Without such an approach, an understanding of persons who are called schizophrenic will at best be truncated and at worst, plainly false.

DISCUSSION

Do you think psychiatry can ever hope for a harmonious marriage between the two positions you outline?

This goal is quite problematical. There is considerable tension between the seeming mutual exclusiveness of the two positions because it appears that you have to choose sides. That tension, however, is not necessary. For example, while we do not have very much difficulty, scientifically, in saying that, for example, a table is more space than matter, we do not just walk through the table; we walk around it. We are comfortable with what might be called the manifest image of the table, as well as with its ultimate scientific image. In this case the reason is that presumably there are not psychological issues tied to the question; there are no "narcissistic" elements to the holding of one position or the other. So perhaps there is the possibility of a marriage, or if you will, a reconciliation, but only if the sources of the antagonism can be made manifest.

Perhaps the positions you outline, and their differences, are not only of conceptual importance but also arise out of the political and social place of psychiatry.

I agree very much. As a matter of fact, I think that there are far fewer scientific determinants of these points of view than there are sociological, ethical, and even aesthetic ones. For example, recall Copernicus. The major difference between him and Ptolemny was that he put the sun, rather than the earth, at the center of the universe. Copernicus kept everything revolving in circles in the same plane, which is not true. He even kept epicycles. His reasons for this were theological. Now I think that psychiatry has a tremendous need these days to maintain itself within the orbit of medicine; it is trying to do this by presenting a kind of scientific posture which, as I have already pointed out, is conceptually naive. It seems to me that in doing so it sacrifices a tremendous dimension of its meaning and its existence. I think it is a very serious problem and can be seen clearly along sociological and ethical lines.

I want to ask you about the issue of the openness to scientific scrutiny of concepts such as intentionality or affective state. For example, take the uniqueness of each psychotherapeutic experience and the question of whether or not it can then be studied "scientifically." I wonder if you would comment on, in your terms, the role of explanation when studying understanding.

It seems to me that the question here is, "What is scientific scrutiny?" Quine says that the only knowledge we need to concern ourselves with is the kind of scientific knowledge that is modeled after the natural sciences. There are problems with this stance, however, in psychiatry. For one thing, psychiatry understands very little, relatively speaking, of the relation between behavior and neurological states. Thus, we do not have the luxury of being able to abandon our everyday view of humanity because we do not yet have the knowledge necessary to do so. But in addition perhaps we do not want to buy the notion that *that* understanding— the physical scientific dimension—is all there is. We may want to say to somebody: "I want to understand you in terms of what has meaning to you. I do not care that there are many people who say that meanings are not measurable or if they are measurable then they are inherently vague. That is the way I want to deal with you and that need is not simply a psychological need." It is a kind of felt need that is related to the way in which we are embodied in the world.

Taking that stance, I am not disturbed by the fact that tensions, feelings, and the like are much harder to measure. In fact I think that they are not the sorts of things that we can measure. Actually, outside of the pure physical sciences, scientific methodology was first applied not in the social sciences but in subjects such as geology and meteorology. Significant problems are encountered in both spheres. There are some principles intrinsic to geology, such as hereditary mechanics, that have to be employed before geology makes sense in any sort of autonomous way. So there is this kind of naive notion that all we have to do is to take the scientific methodology of physics and statistical mechanics and move it over to the sphere of human affairs. That is an enormous leap, conceptually. I think that this is a most difficult move and the burden of proof is upon the shoulders of those people who do it to show that it is useful.

Are you arguing that there are psychological phenomena not understandable with the scientific method?

I raised the Copernicus issue to illustrate that there were theological influences on his conceptions. Nevertheless, his model of the solar system represented a tremendous explanatory advance in understanding, for example, the retrograde motion of Mars or the orbit of Mercury. The issue here is that of instrumentalism versus realism. Are our conceptions of atoms and molecules merely instruments for explanation or do these terms actually denote specific constituents of reality? It is my view and the view of many other philosophers of science that these are not mere instruments but real parts of the world. It is a real entity that we cannot see. We are saying that the capacity to see something ought not to be the ultimate criterion for its existence.

I might say that behind this is an argument that has raged in academic philosophy for over twenty years. The argument is this: On the one hand we have science, which has done the best and the worst for us. It has given us electricity and automobiles as well as atom bombs. It is responsible for both the glories and the horrors of our existence. On the other hand we have the everyday world. Can we find a way of discussing this everyday world that is refined but is still short of being highly technical and scientific? Of course we can—we do that, for example, when we tell somebody about a myocardial infarction. We do not want to talk down to them, so we take a position in between. We do not have to talk about hypercoaguability or atherosclerotic placques, and so on. They would not understand that. At the same time, we do not want to just say "your heart gave out." We can use something called a "model," which scientists do all the time. We tell them that arteries are like tubes and tubes get clogged up and that is exactly what happened to one of their major arteries. Therefore, their blood supplies to the heart became deficient and a heart attack resulted. That is in between a highly theoretical discussion and a silly everyday explanation which would really not account for the events adequately.

What I am saying is that we do not have to be such ultimate theorists that we do away with our everyday view. If we do that, we change ourselves because, as I have said, the very way we are is constituted partly of the way we perceive ourselves to be. If we perceive ourselves merely as atoms, molecules, and the like, then we change what we are. If we do not regard ourselves as agents, as persons who make decisions, then we abandon the manifest image of ourselves to a scientific image and lose a whole dimension of our existence. On the other hand, we do not want to abandon the scientific image of ourselves. What we want to do is to try and find a way in which both these images can be fitted to each other. The way in which I see them fitting together is that the manifest image of man actually is what gives meaning to the scientific image. We will not know what the molecules and electrons are all about with respect to man if we do not know what we mean by an everyday vision of the human being. That is, really, the message of this essay. It is very difficult to make this point; I do not mean just to say that we must treat body and mind together or "treat the whole person." Those concepts may do more harm than good because they are guilty of reifying mental processes and making them what they are not.

Could one not argue that an "everyday" language is merely the result of uneducational bias—that with proper education we could adopt a scientific view, for example, as we now are trying to convert people to the metric system?

Paul Feyerabend adopts that point of view. For instance, in prerelativity physics we thought that things could go as fast as we wanted them to go or that there really was something called mass. We now think postrelativistically, and we are comfortable with these things not being true. Feyerabend's view is that we do have to start talking about atoms and molecules and we have to refine our language as we go along. We have to dispense with ordinary everyday images because they are wrong. All it requires, really, is a reorientation from the time kids start school; we have to teach them to think more molecularly. It will not be such an issue for them, and things like values and the like will no longer exist as they seem to exist right now. Concepts such as values, Feyerabend argues, are examples of conceptually confused problems that are really not very important at all.

I am disagreeing with such a position. It seems to me that the phenomenology and structure of our everyday experience demands that we have the kinds of accounts of ourselves that we provide in an everyday way and that we will not be able to accomplish the kind of behavioral reorganization that he wants. I would hold to the view that Aristotle presents. He says let us take a look at the subject matter, human beings. We cannot hope for a degree of precision that exceeds the complexity of our subject matter. We are not dealing with discrete bodies that move in parabolic paths but rather with a much more complex system. Hence the level of precision we can achieve will be different, and we have to tolerate different methodologies. That is really the message I am trying to get across; not that we cannot have a systematic or a much broader scientific understanding of persons and of processes such as schizophrenia but that such understanding will not simply be modeled after traditional methodologies of physical science.

REFERENCES

Anscombe, G. E. M. 1957. *Intention.* Ithaca: Cornell University Press.

Bastian, H. C. 1898. *A treatise on aphasia and other speech defects.* London: H. K. Lewis.

Braithwaite, R. B. 1953. *Scientific exploration.* Cambridge: Cambridge University Press.

Brentano, F. 1874. *Psychologie vom Empirischen Standpunkt,* vol. 1. Leipzig: Dunker and Humbolt.

Bridgman, P. W. 1927. *The logic of modern physics.* New York: Macmillan.

Chisholm, R. 1957. *Perceiving.* Ithaca: Cornell University Press.

Comte, A. 1853. *The positive philosophy of Auguste Comte.* Ed. H. Martineau. London.

Dilthey, W. 1959. The understanding of other persons and their life-expressions. In *Theories of history: readings in classical and contemporary sources,* ed. P. Gardiner. New York: Free Press.

Droysen, J. G. 1925. *Grundriss der Historik.* Ed. Erich Rothaker. Halle: Max Niesmeyer.

Duhem, P. 1962. *The aim and stature of scientific theory.* New York: Atheneum.

Eddington, A. 1949. *The philosophy of physical science*. Cambridge: Cambridge University Press.

Ellenberger, H. F. 1970. *The discovery of the unconscious*. New York: Basic Books.

Feyerabend, P. 1963. How to be a good empiricist: a plea for tolerance in matters epistomological. In *Philosophy of science: the Delaware Seminar*, vol. 2, ed. B. Baumrin. New York: Wiley.

Flint, R. 1876. Critical notice of *Psychologie vom Empirisohen Standpunkt* by F. Brentano. *Mind* 1:116–122.

Frank, P. 1957. *Philosophy of science*. Englewood Cliffs: Prentice-Hall.

Freud, S. 1897. The project for a scientific psychology. In *The complete psychological works of Sigmund Freud*, vol. 1, ed. J. Strachey. London: Hogarth Press.

_____. 1900. The interpretation of dreams. In *The complete psychological works of Sigmund Freud*, vols. 4 and 5, ed. J. Strachey. London: Hogarth Press.

_____. 1960. *Letters of Sigmund Freud*. Ed. E. L. Freud. New York: Basic Books.

Geschwind, N. 1965a Disconnection syndromes in animals and men, part 1. *Brain* 88:237–274.

_____. 1965b. Disconnection syndrome in animals and men, part 2. *Brain* 88:585–644.

Goldstein, K. 1948. *Language and Language Disturbances*. New York: Grune and Stratton.

Harré, H., and P. F. Secord. 1973. *The explanation of human behavior*. New Jersey: Littlefield, Adams.

Havens, L. 1973. *Approaches to the mind*. Boston: Little, Brown.

Hempel, K. 1942. The function of general laws in history. *Journal of Philosophy* 39:35–48.

_____. 1966. *Philosophy of natural science*. Englewood Cliffs: Prentice-Hall.

Hook, E. B. 1973. Behavioral implications of the human XYY genotype. *Science* 179:139–150.

Jackson, J. H. 1958. *Selected writings of John Hughlings Jackson*, vol. 7. Ed. J. Taylor. New York: Basic Books.

James, W. 1950. *The Principle of psychology*, vols. 1 and 2. New York: Dover.

Kraepelin, E. 1915. *Clinical psychiatry: a textbook for students and physicians*. New York: Macmillan.

_____. 1968. *Lectures on clinical psychiatry*. New York: Hafner.

Land, J. P. N. 1876. Brentano's logical innovations. *Mind* 1:289–292.

Lucia, A. R. 1970. *Traumatic aphasia: its syndromes and treatment*. Paris: Mouton.

Mach, E. 1893. *The science of mechanics: a critical and historic account of its development*. Trans. T. McCormack. LaSalle, Ill.: Open Court.

MacLean, P. D. 1952. Some psychiatric implications of physiological studies on fronto temporal portion of limbic system (visceral brain). *Electroencephalography and Clinical Neurophysiology* 4:407.

Nagel, E. 1951. Mechanistic explanation and organismic biology. *Philosophy and Phenomenological Research* 2:327–338.

_____. 1961. *The structure of science*. New York: Harcourt, Brace and World.

Papez, J. 1937. A proposed mechanism of emotion. *Archives of Neurology and Psychiatry* 38:725–743.

Popper, K. 1962. *The open society and its enemies*, vol. 2. New York: Harper and Row.

Quine, W. V. 1960. *Word and object*. Cambridge: MIT Press.

_____. 1970. *The web of belief*. New York: Random House.

Rapaport, D. 1960. The structure of psychoanalytic theory. *Psychological issues* 6.

Rickert, H. 1926. *Kulturwissenschaft und Naturwissenschaft*, 5th ed. Tubingen: J. C. B. Mohr.

Rosenbluth, A., N. Wiener, and J. Bigelow. 1943. Behavior, purpose and teleology. *Philosophy of Science* 10:18–24.

Russell, B. 1959. *My philosophical development*. London: Allen and Unwin.

Schuldenfrei, R. 1972. Quine in perspective. *Journal of Philosophy* 69: 5–16.

Sellars, W. 1963. *Science, Perception and Reality*. New York: Humanities Press.

Skinner, B. F. 1972. *Cumulative record: a selection of papers*. New York: Appleton-Century-Crofts.

Slater, E., and V. Cowie. 1971. *The genetics of mental disorders*. London: Oxford University Press.

Stebbing, L. S. 1937. *Philosophy and the physicists*. London: Methnen.

Taylor, C. 1964. *The explanation of behavior*. New York: Humanities Press.

Von Wright, G. H. 1971. *Explanation and understanding*. Ithaca: Cornell University Press.

Weber, M. 1949. *On the methodology of the social sciences*. Trans. and ed. E. A. Shils and H. A. Finch. Glencoe: Free Press.

Woodruff, R. A., D. W. Goodwin, and S. B. Guze. 1974. *Psychiatric diagnosis*. New York: Oxford University Press.

PART TWO

Etiology:
The Nature-Nurture
Interaction

3

Heredity and Environment

SEYMOUR KETY

Many years ago, when I lived in Philadelphia and Toscanini was guest conductor of the Philadelphia Orchestra, the story was told that during a rehearsal Toscanini noticed the concert master making faces. Stopping suddenly, Toscanini said, "You don't like my conducting?" To which the concert master replied, "Oh, Maestro, you are the greatest. I love your conducting. You are perfect." So they started again, and again the concert master made faces, and Toscanini said, "Perhaps you don't like Beethoven?" "Oh, Beethoven, Beethoven is the greatest composer of all." So they started again, and the concert master continued to make faces. At that point Toscanini became very angry and said, "I insist—tell me why you are making faces like that. You said it was not because you don't like me, and it's not because you don't like Beethoven." The concert master finally replied, "It's just that I don't like music!"

Now there are some people who just don't like genetics. For a long time genetics was in disrepute because of the assumption that if something was genetic in nature you could not do anything about it; it was fixed and immutable. Today, with the vaguest hint that it may be possible to alter "genetic determination," it is again the object of attack—but now because of "genetic manipulation."

In psychiatry there has always been evidence to suggest the operation of genetic factors in the major mental illnesses, evidence which had many shortcomings but which was nevertheless difficult to ignore. Schizophrenia and manic depressive psychosis was observed to run in families. There is a ten percent risk for schizophrenia in the first-degree relatives of schizophrenics and a one percent risk for schizophrenia in the general population. Then there were the twin studies in which it was shown repeatedly (in more than twelve studies) that the monozygotic twin of a schizophrenic or manic depressive patient is much more likely to have the same illness than is a dizygotic twin. In fact, the risk for schizophrenia in the co-twin of a dizygotic schizophrenic is about ten percent, the same as for other siblings. In a monozygotic twin, on the other hand, the risk is fifty percent.

Such evidence, however, was not accepted as proof that genetic factors are important in these illnesses, and for good reasons. There were fairly large loopholes in this evidence—large enough for whole schools of psychiatry to march through them. What was the difficulty? Even though schizophrenia runs in families, many things run in families. Poverty runs in families, wealth runs in families, pellagra runs in families. That is hardly good evidence that these are genetically determined, since families share not only genetic endowment but also environment and life experience. Therefore, showing that something runs in families proves very little about its origins.

Twin studies are a more compelling form of genetic data, but even twin studies depend on the assumption that the only thing that differentiates monozygotic from dizygotic twins is their genetic relatedness, and that environmental factors are somehow canceled out or randomized. But that is not the case. Monozygotic twins share much of their environment as well as their genetic endowment. They live together; they sleep together; they are dressed alike by their parents; they are paraded in a double parambulator as infants; their friends can not distinguish one from the other. In short, they develop a certain ego identification with each other that is very hard to dissociate from the purely genetic identity with which they were born.

It was interpretive difficulties such as these that in 1961 stimulated several of us at the National Institute of Mental Health—David Rosenthal, Paul Wender, and myself—to decide independently that there was another approach to the problem of dissociating genetic from environmental variables in schizophrenia.

We reasoned that although an adopted person derives his genetic endowment from one family, his life experience and environment occur with another family. This occurred to me because I noticed a rather interesting peculiarity of adoptive parents. Such parents notice various characteristics in their adopted child and have a tendency to attribute to genetic factors the qualities they do not like about the child; on the other hand, if the child does things of which they approve, they attribute them to their environment. That, of course, is wishful thinking, but it did suggest the possibility of separating the two influences by a more scientific process. We also realized that to avoid selective bias, it would be necessary to start with a total population of adoptive individuals and then identify those who were schizophrenic rather than to start with schizophrenics and try to find those who were adopted. To avoid subjective bias all diagnoses would have to be made in ignorance of the relationship of one individual to another.

After trying in the United States to pull together a total sample, we gave up and went to Denmark. We were given access, on the basis of complete confidentiality, to the remarkably accurate records that Denmark keeps on its inhabitants. An adoption file has all of the country's legally adopted individuals going back for a number of generations. Because we were interested only in adoptees who were adults at the time of the study and therefore old enough to have acquired schizophrenia, we searched for mental illness among the 14,500 people in Denmark who are now between twenty-five and fifty years of age and who were legally adopted at an early age by people other than their biological relatives. Because Denmark has a system of national health insurance, there is also a central register that lists the names of all people who have been seen in any psychiatric facility in Denmark, with the exception of one hospital, which for a long time refused to report. We therefore made a search through the psychiatric register and, separately, through the records of that one hospital. We found that the psychiatric register was quite complete; by going through the hospital records individually we found that only five percent of the people ever admitted to a mental hospital were not listed in the register. We therefore searched through the register for any one of those 14,500 adoptees who had ever been seen in a psychiatric facility. Ten percent of then had—about what one would expect in the general population in Denmark.

The difficult problem then arose of picking out those who could be called schizophrenic, since schizophrenia means different things in different places. In Denmark, schizophrenia is what Kraepelin thought it was, that is, chronic process schizophrenia. But in America other subgroups have been added to the original syndrome. There is a category of latent, ambulatory, or borderline schizophrenia that has many of the characteristics of chronic schizophrenia except that it usually does not have the psychotic features. Another category, called acute schizophrenic reaction, is simply an acute psychotic reaction that in Denmark would be called schizophreniform psychosis or psychogenic psychosis but would not be called schizophrenia. We decided that since American psychiatry calls all three categories schizophrenia we would, for the purpose of our study, accept all three, but would define each category appropriately and use the diagnoses carefully in the hope that we might find out not only whether genetic factors operate but also what different factors operate in these different categories of schizophrenia.

We read the psychiatric records or abstracts, translated into English, of those adoptees who had been seen in a psychiatric facility. By this time the three of us had established a collaboration with Fini Schulsinger, who is Chief of Psychiatry at the Kommunehospital and through whose good offices we had been introduced to the record system in Denmark and to the authorities. Schulsinger organized a team in Denmark to collect the data that we required.

If the three of us in America and Schulsinger independently agreed that someone was schizophrenic in one of the three categories, then that perosn became an index case. If we all four independently decided he was not schizophrenic, then he was rejected. If one or another of us suggested schizophrenia, then we would hold a conference on that particular case and if as a result of that conference we could all agree on schizophrenia, then he would become an index case. In this way, we selected seventy-four persons whom we all finally diagnosed as schizophrenia. What we wanted to do was to examine their biological and adoptive relatives; if schizophrenia runs in the family because of shared environmental factors, it should run in the adoptive families, whereas if the familial tendency in schizophrenia is the result of heredity, it would appear in the biological relatives. In Denmark it is not difficult to identify the relatives of adoptive persons: the adoption records themselves are quite complete, giving the names of biological parents and adoptive parents, and there is a register listing the name of anyone who has lived in Denmark more than three weeks, his birthdate, all addresses he has had since birth, the names of every child in the household, name of spouse, and so forth. By going through this register with the names of the parents, biological and adoptive, we could identify all the other children the parents had. These children would then be full siblings or half siblings of the adoptee, depending upon whether they shared both parents or only one. In this manner we assembled the relatives of the seventy-four index adoptees with schizophrenia, as well as the relatives of seventy-four adopted controls, each matched with an index case in terms of age, sex, socioeconomic class of the rearing family, and length of time spent with the biological mother.

We then shuffled these names together and from then on we identified relatives and made diagnoses without knowing the relationship of one person to another or whether the person was related to an index case or control. The total of index cases and controls gave us more than 1,100 relatives. The names of these relatives were then searched through the psychiatric register as well as other registers—for example, military records and records compiled by the Department of Justice from psychiatric examinations of prisoners. In all such sources we looked for relatives who had had any experience with a psychiatrist or a psychiatric institution. That information was abstracted, translated into English, and edited to remove any clues that would permit a sophisticated reader to guess whether this was a biological relative, an adoptive relative, an index or control relative. Then each of us independently read these records and made a psychiatric diagnosis using the three types of schizophrenia that we were tentatively accepting: chronic, borderline or latent, and acute. We quickly decided that we needed to create another category, questionable or uncertain schizophrenia. In picking the index cases, we had excluded those in which the schizophrenia was uncertain, but with the relatives we had to make a diagnosis, even if we were not sure. Thus, "uncertain schizophrenia" included those cases in which the symptoms were too mild or atypical for a diagnosis or in which for some reason or another we thought schizophrenia was the most likely diagnosis but could not be sure. As a result, we were testing the hypothesis that genetic factors in schizophrenia might be manifested not only in the three kinds of schizophrenia we had labeled but also in cases of uncertain schizophrenia. For some time there has been the notion that "schizoid" or "inadequate" personality disorder is also a *forme fruste* of schizophrenia. We speculated that there might be a schizophrenic spectrum of disorders that ranged from definite schizophrenia through these types of uncertain schizophrenia. If we could get enough information, we hoped that we would be able to test this hypothesis.

When we had diagnosed all relatives on whom we had any information, we broke the code and allocated the relatives to their respective populations. What we found was as follows: Among the index cases, 24 out of 405 biological relatives exhibited a schizophrenic spectrum disorder, whereas 2 out of 173 adoptive relatives exhibited these disorders. Among the control cases, 4 out of 387 biological relatives and 4 out of 194 adoptive relatives exhibited a schizophrenic spectrum disorder. The difference in schizophrenic spectrum disorders between index and control biologic relatives is highly significant ($p=0.0001$). The number of schizophrenic spectrum disorders in the biologic and adoptive relatives of the controls and in the adoptive relatives of the index cases are the one or two percent that one would expect in the population as a whole. On the other hand, the biological relatives of index cases show a significant concentration of spectrum disorders, nearly six percent.

Table 3.1 separates the biological relatives of the index cases according to the diagnosis we made in each index case. Of the 74 index cases, 37 had received a diagnosis of chronic Kraepelinian schizophrenia; of their 217 biological relatives, 16 have some schizophrenic diagnosis: 6 chronic, 6 latent, 4 uncertain schizophrenia. Thus, there is a significant concentration of chronic schizophrenia in the biological relatives of chronic schizophren-

Table 3.1. Definite (chronic or borderline) and uncertain schizophrenia in the biological relatives of the schizophrenic adoptee, according to the diagnosis of the adoptee.

Diagnosis of adoptee	Adoptees diagnosed	Biological relatives				
		Chronic	Latent	Uncertain	Total diagnosed	Total identified
Chronic	37	6	6	4	16	217
Acute	13	0	0	0	0	61
Latent	24	1	3	1	5	128

ics, as well as a significant prevalence of a less severe form. This certainly suggests that latent and uncertain schizophrenia have some genetic relation to classical Kraepelinian schizophrenia. By contrast, of the 13 index cases who were diagnosed as having acute schizophrenic reaction, none of their biological relatives had schizophrenia. This is certainly compatible with what many investigators have suspected: that the illnesses of patients who have an acute psychotic break for the first time and do not go on to more chronic schizophrenic illness are more related to the affective disorders than to schizophrenia. George Vaillant went back over records at the Massachusetts Mental Health Center of the families of people with acute schizophrenic reaction and found that there were a lot of affective disorders and relatively little schizophrenia (Vaillant 1962). Perhaps every acute psychotic break should not be labeled schizophrenia but should rather be diagnosed as an acute psychotic reaction of unknown etiology. The 24 latent schizophrenic adoptees had some chronic, some latent, and some uncertain schizophrenia in their biological relatives. This suggests again that latent or borderline schizophrenia, in contrast to "acute schizophrenia," may be related to process schizophrenia as Kraepelin described it. Recently Spitzer and Endicott have independently made diagnoses on a subsample of these probands and relatives, confirming our diagnoses of chronic schizophrenia and finding a high prevalence of schizophrenia and a less severe syndrome (which they have designated "schizotypal personality" instead of "latent" or "uncertain" schizophrenia) in their biological relatives.

Now what about environmental factors? All that we could say was that the data suggested the operation of genetic factors, but that did not exclude environmental factors, even though the adoptive relatives did not show any more schizophrenia than the adoptive relatives of controls. We therefore thought that it would be useful if we could carry out intensive psychiatric interviews with these relatives. This might give us a great deal more information about their mental status, personalities, and environmental influences. Such interviews might also make possible psychiatric diagnoses on people who had never been seen by a psychiatrist. It was clearly impractical to conduct interviews on all 1,100 relatives. However, we felt that we could do such a study on a subgroup of this population, the subgroup that were adopted in greater Copenhagen (Kety et al., 1975). Of the 14,500 adoptees, 5,500 were adopted through the courts of Copenhagen, and of these 5,500, 33 were among our index cases and 33 were among the controls. These individuals had given us 512 of the 1,100 relatives.

We were very fortunate to enlist the collaboration of Bjørn Jacobsen, a young psychiatrist who spent two years carrying out these interviews. There were, of course, some ethical considerations in such an enterprise. We had agreed with the authorities that we would keep all the information confidential, even from people whom it might concern. And we did not think it was ethical to go up to a middle-aged housewife in Denmark and say, "Mrs. Hansen, we would like to interview you because at the age of eighteen you had an illegitimate child who now has schizophrenia." On the other hand, we felt that it was necessary to inform prospective subjects regarding the nature of the interview but without discussing adoption, the hypothesis that was being tested, or how they were selected. So we wrote to all the relatives in the greater Copenhagen sample that we were interested in doing a study on factors concerning health and requesting their participation in an interview by a physician regarding their life history and its medical-psychological aspects. They were assured that the interview would be protected by the Danish laws of confidentiality for information given to physicians. These interview have been used only for research and are not available to the Danish system of records.

About half the people immediately responded, giving a time when the interview could take place. Those that did not respond got a telephone call from the secretary first and then from Jacobsen, who tried to persuade them. For those who still had not responded, Jacobsen would knock on their door and try to persuade them to have an interview. In this way ninety percent of the relatives alive and residing in Denmark, Sweden, or Norway agreed to an interview.

The interviews were exhaustive, averaging thirty-five pages in transcript. They elicited a great deal of medical, psychological, and sociological information on the individual from birth, as well as providing a complete mental status examination. The interviews were dictated by Jacobsen in English and edited to remove any clues identifying the biological or adoptive relationship of the person to our index or control cases. Rosenthal, Wender, and myself then again read and classified each interview. Schulsinger did not participate in this step because we thought he might know some of the people in the Copenhagen sample.

Table 3.2 shows the status of the relatives when we completed the study. First, there was a very significant increase in deaths among the biological relatives of the index group, thirty-five as compared to thirteen in the control group. We tracked down the causes of death in most of these cases through death certificates and hospital records and found that the excess of death was accounted for by suicide or probable suicide and a few other kinds of sudden death. When we counted only natural deaths or medical illnesses, the numbers in each group were comparable. In fact, all of the eight suicides in the total population of relatives were biological relatives of the index group. Since suicide is an unfortunate outcome in many instances of schizophrenia, it is possible that some schizophrenics had removed themselves from our sample before they were ever diagnosed as such.

Table 3.3 shows our diagnoses of psychiatric disorders outside the schizophrenia spectrum. There were fewer index biological relatives interviewed because of the higher death rate among them. The percentages shown are the percentages of relatives that were interviewed. We considered about forty percent of the relatives to be normal, or at least without a psychiatric diagnosis,

Table 3.2. Interview status of relatives.[a]

Relatives	Identified	Died	Emigrated beyond Scandinavia	Disappeared (or institutionalized)	Refused interview	Refused interview; gave no information
Biological relatives of index group	173	35	13	1 (1)	12	6
Biological relatives of control group	174	13	11	1	11	9
Adoptive relatives of index group	74	35	0	0	5	4
Adoptive relatives of control group	91	36	2	1	7	4
Total	512	119	26	4	35	23

[a] All differences between index and control groups are nonsignificant except for deaths between index and control groups of biological relatives ($p < 0.001$, Fischer's exact probability, one-tailed).

and these were distributed randomly. In about fifty percent of the relatives we made some type of psychiatric diagnosis, and these diagnoses also seemed to be randomly distributed.

For schizophrenia diagnoses, however, the situation is different: eight percent of the biological relatives of the index group were given the diagnosis of definite schizophrenia, and one to three percent of the control relatives, a highly significant difference (table 3.4). If we add to that the people we called uncertain schizophrenics (table 3.5), we simply get an exaggeration of the same phenomenon: now we have definite or uncertain schizophrenia in sixteen percent of those who are genetically related to the index cases. Thus, uncertain schizophrenics also cluster in the biological relatives of the index cases.

Table 3.3. Consensus diagnoses outside the schizophrenia spectrum in biological and adoptive relatives.

Relatives	Number outside of spectrum	Psychiatrically normal	All nonspectrum diagnoses	Organic	Neurotic	Affective	Personality
Biological relatives of index group	81	37%	49%	9%	5%	2%	33%
Biological relatives of control group	121	41%	51%	5%	5%	9%	32%
Adoptive relatives of index group	31	36%	55%	16%	10%	3%	26%
Adoptive relatives of control group	41	27%	63%	15%	5%	7%	37%

Table 3.4. Definite schizophrenia (chronic or borderline[a]) in all identified relatives (512).[b]

Relatives	Identified	Having definite schizophrenia	Percent
Biological relatives of index group	173	14	8.1
Biological relatives of control group	174	4	2.3
Adoptive relatives of index group	74	1	1.4
Adoptive relatives of control group	91	3	3.3

[a] Acute schizophrenia was not found in the relatives.
[b] The difference between index and control groups in biological relatives is significant at $p = 0.013$.

Table 3.5. Definite or uncertain schizophrenia in all identified relatives (512).[a]

Relatives	Identified	Having definite or uncertain schizophrenia	Percent
Biological relatives of index group	173	28	16.2
Biological relatives of control group	174	8	4.6
Adoptive relatives of index group	74	3	4.1
Adoptive relatives of control group	91	6	6.6

[a] The difference between index and control groups in biological relatives is significant at $p = 0.0003$.

Table 3.6 includes relatives whom we regarded as falling somewhere in the areas of schizoid or inadequate personality. Here we did not find a significant difference. Seven and one half percent of the biological relatives of the index group versus seven and one half percent of their controls were called inadequate or schizoid personality. The smaller percentages in the adoptive relatives can probably be ascribed not to more psychopathology in biological relatives of adoptees but to an age difference. Thus, this study does not provide evidence that schizoid personality is a form of schizophrenia.

There is a major loophole in all of this evidence, however. Adoption does not separate genetic from environmental factors completely, because even an adopted child shares an environment *in utero* with his biological mother and receives a certain amount of early mothering at her hands. It is not impossible that during perinatal period some environmental factors could be transmitted from the mother to the child which, twenty years later, might result in schizophrenia. We approached this problem in the following way: There are a lot of biological half siblings in this sample because the biological parents usually were not married at the time they had the child they put up for adoption, and

Table 3.6. Inadequate or schizoid personality in all identified relatives (512).

Relatives	Identified	Having inadequate or schizoid personality	Percent
Biological relatives of index group	173	13	7.5
Biological relatives of control group	174	13	7.5
Adoptive relatives of index group	74	2	2.7
Adoptive relatives of control group	91	2	2.2

many subsequently had other children with their partners. And since a man can have more children in a given period of time than a woman can, we found as expected that the fathers had substantial numbers of children with other partners; these would be the biological paternal half siblings of our adoptees, of whom there were 127—more than any other type of relative in the sample. Paternal half siblings help us with this problem because they have the same father but different mothers, that is, they do not share the same uterine environment or the same early mothering experience. Table 3.7 shows data for these paternal half siblings. There are a nearly equal number in each group, sixty-three biological paternal half siblings of the index cases, sixty-four of the controls. The amount of schizophrenia, however, is very heavily concentrated in the index relatives. In the case of definite or uncertain schizophrenia, twenty-two percent of the biological paternal half siblings of the schizophrenic adoptees have this diagnosis, versus three percent of the controls; if we restrict ourselves to definite schizophrenia, it is thirteen percent versus two percent—differences that are highly significant.

We have concluded from these findings that genetic factors must be operating in schizophrenia. But what is the nature of

Table 3.7. Schizophrenia in the biological paternal half siblings of the index and control adoptees.

Adoptee	Identi-fied	Having definite or uncertain schizophrenia[a]	Percent	Having definite schizophrenia[b]	Percent
Index	63	14	22.0	8	13.0
Control	64	2	3.0	1	1.6

[a] Difference is significant at $p = 0.001$.
[b] Difference is significant at $p = 0.015$.

these genetic factors? When we inspected individual families closely, we found some other interesting information. The relatives with chronic schizophrenia were nearly always in the biological families of the chronic schizophrenic adoptees. Secondly, the adoptees with borderline schizophrenia never have biological relatives with schizophrenia more severe than borderline. Moreover, no schizophrenia-like illness appeared in the biological relatives of half of the adoptees. This suggests that we may be dealing not with a single illness but with a heterogeneous cluster of illnesses that have different etiologies.

We also have to recognize the possibility that there are forms of schizophrenia in which genetic loading is very important and forms of schizophrenia in which environmental factors probably play the important role. The best evidence that environmental factors are important comes from twin studies, which show that the concordance rate among monozygotic twins is only fifty percent. Clearly, genetic factors cannot account for the whole story. How, then, to get at the environmental factors? Certainly there has been a great emphasis for the past twenty-five years on intrafamily psychological factors, schizophrenogenic mothers, schizophrenogenic parents, the communication of irrationality, and the like. Theodore Lidz has been a major proponent of this position, which he based on observation and psychoanalytic interviews with the parents of schizophrenics at the Yale Psychiatric Institute (Lidz et al. 1975; see also chapter 4 of this book). Lidz finds a high incidnce of psychopathology in parents of schizophrenic patients, to which he attributes an etiological role in the schizophrenia of the children. It seems to me, however, that there are a number of loopholes in his evidence regarding schizophrenogenic parents, as sensitive and perceptive as it is. There are no controls, for example, and the interviewers were not blind. It is difficult to see how an interviewer could avoid finding what he expected to find, given the complexity and the enormous amount of data in a series of psychoanalytic interviews.

Alanen, recognizing the need for controls, compared the parents of schizophrenics with those of neurotics and normal individuals (Alanen 1966). Alanen was not entirely blind, and therefore his observations suffer from a certain amount of subjective bias. Nonetheless, he found much more psychopathology in the parents of schizophrenics than in the parents of neurotics, who in turn had more psychopathology than the parents of normal individuals. More recently, Wynne and Singer have been carrying out a number of studies in which a great effort is made to control the observations (Wynne et al. 1976). Their studies depend largely on projective tests, especially the Rorschach. Rorschach testing is done with parents by an observer who may or may not be blind, but then the tapes of these interviews are sent to Margaret Singer, who analyzes them without knowing whether the subjects are related to schizophrenics or controls. Using this method, Wynne and Singer report not so much frank psychopathology as consistent "communication deviance."

There are, however, three alternative hypotheses that such studies have not ruled out. One possibility is that parental differences, including deviant communication, could be a reflection of genetic factors that the parents share with their schizophrenic offspring. A second hypothesis is that the problems associated with rearing a schizophrenic child do something to parents— change them psychologically, alter their pattern of communication in some way. A third alternative is that there is some artifact in the testing situation: someone who has reared a schizophrenic may react differently during psychological testing from someone who has not had that experience. That hypothesis has some interesting support from work by Shopler and Loftin (1969). They tested one group of parents of psychotic children after telling them that they were doing so to learn more about the illness in their child. Another group of parents were tested after being told that they had reared a normal child (which they had); the fact that they had also reared a psychotic child was ignored. The parents presumably took the test situation with the two different sets; only one group had a feeling that they were being studied because of the schizophrenia in their child. More psychopathology was found in the parents who were told that the test's purpose was to learn about their psychotic child. So it is quite possible that the guilt feelings and anxieties of parents of schizophrenics might cause differences that a sophisticated observer could detect in the parents' responses to projective tests.

Wender thought it was possible to test some of these hypotheses by using the adoption model, so he pulled together a population of adopted schizophrenics in Bethesda (Wender et al. 1968; 1971). This was a sample of Americans whose adoptive parents were alive and would stay at the Clinical Center in Bethesda long enough for them and their schizophrenic sons or daughters to be studied. Psychiatric evaluation, Rorschach tests, and other kinds of projective tests were performed. Similar assessments were carried out on a group of adoptive parents of normal children and on a group of natural parents of schizophrenics who had reared their own children. When psychopathology in the parents was classified according to Alanen's system, as much psychopathology was found in the natural parents of schizophrenics as Alanen had found. On the other hand, the adoptive parents of schizophrenics had less psychopathology, about as much as Alanen had found in the parents of neurotics. This is similar to our finding in the Danish sample that the adoptive parents of schizophrenics consistently showed no more schizophrenia and no more psychopathology in general than do the adoptive parents of controls.

Wender sent the Rorschach tapes of these parents to Margaret Singer for her blind analysis. She came up with a very interesting result (Wynne et al. 1976). With one hundred percent accuracy she could differentiate parents who had reared a schizophrenic from those who had reared a normal individual, whether or not the schizophrenic was genetically related to the parents. In other words, she found some kind of communication deviance in all of the people who had reared a schizophrenic. Now that excludes one hypothesis—the hypothesis that what Wynne and Singer have been measuring is simply a reflection of the genetic overlap between the parents and the offspring. But what does it really mean? One interpretation is that now at last one has proven that communication deviance is of etiologic significance in schizophrenia. A more precise conclusion, however, would be that people who have reared a schizophrenic give different responses in a Rorschach test than do those who have not. The possibility that having reared a schizophrenic affects the psychology of the parents or their response to a test situation has still not been ruled out.

Wender has gone on to do another Rorschach study comparing the adopted parents of schizophrenics, the biological parents of schizophrenics, and the parents of children with a nongenetic form of mental retardation (Wender et al. 1977). In this comparison it was not possible to differentiate the parents of schizophrenics from the parents of mentally retarded individuals, although both groups were different from the normals. This is compatible with the thesis that rearing any seriously disturbed child may change the response of a parent to a projective test and make it possible for sophisticated observers to differentiate them from parents who have not had that experience. The possibility that rearing or particular aspects of rearing are etiologically important in schizophrenia is viable and certainly worth examining further, but it is a hypothesis to be tested rather than an established fact.

What other factors might be operating in the environmental sphere? In our Danish interviews we obtained much information about the background of the relatives that has now been coded, and John Rimmer has been carrying out an extensive computer analysis of the data. He is seeking to define some factors that distinguish adoptive relatives of schizophrenics from adoptive relatives of the controls. No consistent feature has as yet been distinguished, but this approach may be relatively insensitive. Psychoanalytic interviews probably obtain more information than Jacobsen did in his psychiatric examination of only a few hours. The mere fact that we have been unable to find a systematic pattern of differences does not rule out the possibility of their existence.

A couple of years ago Dennis Kinney asked me whether he

could work on our adoption data with a very ingenious approach. Recalling that half of the schizophrenic adoptees had schizophrenic biological relatives while half did not, he pointed out that those adoptees who became schizophrenic with relatively little genetic predisposition would constitute a good sample in which to look for important environmental factors. In fact, by comparing the two groups of schizophrenic adoptees, those environmental variables might emerge. Kinney therefore studied these adoptees and their relatives without knowing which adoptee had a genetic load and which did not.

Among the schizophrenic adoptees with a low genetic risk he found a significantly higher incidence of brain injury, either at birth or postnatally. Furthermore, Herbert Barry reported some years ago the interesting finding that there was an excess of schizophrenics born in the cold winter months (Barry and Barry 1964). This prompted other studies, and eventually Dalen (1968), reviewing all the studies in the literature and his own findings in Sweden, concluded that there was a consistent but slight excess of schizophrenics born in winter. Interestingly enough, in our Copenhagen sample of only thirty-three schizophrenics, Kinney has found that eighty percent of the adoptees with low genetic risk were born in the January to April period; the adoptees with medium to high genetic risk showed the normal expectancy of approximately thirty percent of births in the January to April period. Between brain injury and being born in the cold winter months, he can account for every one of the schizophrenic adoptees with a low genetic risk except one, this one being the only adoptee who had an adoptive sibling with chronic schizophrenia.

What does all this mean? Dalen finds that the cold winter months are associated with greater birth trauma. It is also true, however, that there are peaks of certain virus infections during that time as well as in the summer months, which would represent the first trimester of the pregnancies. Kinney concludes that of these thirty-three schizophrenics, all but one are associated with some crucial biological factor, be it genetic predisposition, brain injury, or a seasonal factor than may be birth injury, a viral infection, or something as yet unidentified.

Still there is so much we do not know. We do not know the

mode of genetic transmission. We do not know the biochemical mechanisms by which the genes express themselves. We do not know the environmental factors that are also necessary for schizophrenia. Certainly we have many interesting hypotheses for all these questions, but none of these hypotheses has really been proven. But we are fortunate today in having plausible, heuristic hypotheses and a generation of young investigators motivated and competent to test them.

DISCUSSION

In the second half of your essay you raise some intriguing questions about the nature of schizophrenic illness. Are there perhaps biochemical or physiological classifications that would make more sense than our traditional psychological criteria?

My personal hunch is that schizophrenia is something like mental retardation, a final common pathway for a variety of causative factors. It would not surprise me if we find as we go along that we will be chipping away at the syndrome of schizophrenia. In the biochemical sphere, I know of two instances of schizophrenics who were diagnosed at reputable psychiatric institutions and eventually turned out to have a clear-cut genetic mutant disease. One of these is the case reported by Mudd and Freeman (1975) at Johns Hopkins, who was shown to have a very rare form of homocystinuria. When she was treated with large doses of folic acid, the schizophrenia disappeared only to recur when the folic acid was removed. Three hundred schizophrenics were immediately examined for this illness and not one of them showed the condition, so it is certainly a very rare cause of schizophrenia. In a recent issue of the *American Journal of Psychiatry*, there is a case of an association between a schizophreniform psychosis and albinism (Baron 1976). One could say that these cases are not schizophrenia, but how do you know they are not schizophrenia? They looked schizophrenic enough to competent psychiatrists when the diagnosis was originally made.

Huntington's chorea starts with schizophreniform symptomatology before it becomes a neurological disorder. The first case of Huntington's chorea in a family is usually diagnosed as schizophrenia. There is an adult form of metachromatic leukodystrophy, a very rare, severe, progressive neurological disorder. Only twenty-four cases have been reported, but practically all were diagnosed as schizophrenia before the neurological findings became manifest. Then, of course, we have many viral encephalopathies that look like schizophrenia before they become more general and diffuse in their manifestations. I think it is possible that any of these disorders may effect certain parts of the brain, including, for example, the limbic system and the frontal lobes. Perhaps certain systems in the brain that mediate the psychological manifestations of schizophrenia can be affected by genetic factors, viral agents, toxins, or physical trauma. If the process stops there, we may have schizophrenia. If it goes on and becomes more generalized, we may end up with a more definite neurological picture.

What I am saying is that from the biological point of view there are simply many possible etiologies for schizophrenia. The relation between biological and psychosocial factors is often unclear. Perhaps the biological lesion is capable of producing schizophrenia only when certain kinds of psychosocial experiences occur.

You speak of a similarity, possibly, between schizophrenia and mental retardation. Would chromosome studies then perhaps be important for genetic research in schizophrenia?

There have been cytogenetic studies in schizophrenics, but without very impressive results. There is a higher incidence of chromosomal abnormality in schizophrenia than there is in the normal population, but that higher incidence is in the area of one to two percent. Perhaps these are chromosomal abnormalities like XXY or one of the supernumerary chromosomal disorders that do affect personality enough to result in a diagnosis of schizophrenia. But I am not aware of any clear-cut evidence of consistent chromosomal abnormalities in schizophrenia. There are some newer flourescent techniques that can identify regions of chromosomes with a great deal of accuracy, and it might be worthwhile for somebody to look at the chromosomes of schizophrenics in that way.

You have enunciated very sharply a possible distinction between schizophrenics who have genetic loading and schizophrenics who perhaps do not. I wonder if you have some thoughts about the clinical implications of such a distinction. We put a great deal of effort into treatment of persons with this illness; consider the time, money, and effort that is invested, especially with many chronic schizophrenic persons. Should we look forward to a time when our treatment approach might be different, depending on the presence or absence of genetic loading?

I think that is quite possible. If one could be sure that certain persons have schizophrenia as a result of psychosicial, educational, or rearing factors, one might try to undo that by an appropriate unraveling of the psychosocial processes. But remember that even those who have a low genetic load may have some biological explanation, at least in Dennis Kinney's view. One might still prevent the occurrence of schizophrenia if it requires a particular virus in order to become manifest.

It is important to point out that merely because an illness is "genetic" does not preclude an environmental cure. For example, there is a genetic predisposition to tuberculosis, but we now have nearly one hundred percent control with proper public health conditions and specific antibiotic medication.

I agree, of course. Genetic or biological factors do not necessarily directly produce the disorder. They could produce a predisposition that requires certain types of life experience. That is certainly perfectly plausible—but unproved.

In Dennis Kinney's study, did he look at the outcome of the two groups that are high and low in genetic loading?

That is being done. Kinney and Wender are doing a thorough clinical survey on these groups to see what clinically differentiates the people with the genetic load from those without it.

In your data on the paternal half siblings, how can we be sure that those fathers might not have sought out a schizophrenogenic mate repeatedly?

That is a very good question. Frankly, we cannot rule it out; but this hypothesis requires the assumption that the fathers have some uncanny ability, greater than that of any psychiatrist I know, to pick out schizophrenogenic mothers. Furthermore, if the father had the propensity for picking schizophrenogenic mothers, this still would not be as effective as *being* the schizophrenogenic mother. On the basis of the hypothesis you propose, we would expect the biological maternal half siblings to have more schizophrenia than the paternal half siblings. That is not what we find. Both maternal and paternal half siblings of schizophrenic adoptees have a higher prevalence of schizophrenia, and in fact the prevalence is slightly higher in the paternal half siblings—so this hypothesis receives no support. Somehow, the conclusion that the schizophrenia is the result of genetic factors seems more plausible and parsimonious.

REFERENCES

Alanen, Y. O. 1966. The family in the pathogenesis of schizophrenic and neurotic disorders. *Acta Psychiatrica Scandinavica* 40:189.

Baron, M. 1976. Albinism and schizophreniform psychosis: a pedigree study. *American Journal of Psychiatry* 133(9):1070–1073.

Barry, H. III, and H. Barry, Jr. 1964. Season of birth in schizophrenics: its relation to social class. *Archives of General Psychiatry* 2:385–391.

Dalen, P. 1968. Month of birth and schizophrenia. *Acta Psychiatrica Scandinavica* (supplement) 203:55.

Kety, S. S., D. Rosenthal, P. H. Wender, et al. 1975. Mental illness in the biological and adoptive families of adopted individuals who become schizophrenic: a preliminary report based on psychiatric interviews. In *Genetic research in psychiatry*, ed. R. Fieve, D. Rosenthal, H. Brill. Baltimore: Johns Hopkins University Press.

Lidz, T., S. Fleck, and A. R. Cornelison. 1975. *Schizophrenia and the family.* New York: International Universities Press.

Mudd, S. H., and J. M. Freeman. 1975. N5, 10-methylenetetrahydrofolaxe reductase deficiency and schizophrenia: a working hypothesis. In *Catecholamine and schizophrenia,* ed. S. W. Matthysse and S. S. Kety. Oxford: Pergamon Press.

Rosenthal, D., P. H. Wender, S. S. Kety, et al. 1971. The adopted away offspring of schizophrenics. *American Journal of Psychiatry* 128:307–311.

Schopler E., and J. Loftin. 1969. Thought disorders in parents of psychotic children. *Archives of General Psychiatry* 20:174–181.

Vaillant, G. E. 1962. The prediction of recovery in schizophrenia. *Journal of Nervous Mental Disorders* 135:534–543.

Wender, P. H., D. Rosenthal, and S. S. Kety. 1968. Psychiatric assessment of adoptive parents of schizophrenics. In *The transmission of schizophrenia,* ed. D. Rosenthal and S. S. Kety. Oxford: Pergamon Press.

Wender, P. H., D. Rosenthal, S. S. Kety, et al. 1974. Crossfostering: a research strategy for clarifying the role of genetic and experiential factors in the etiology of schizophrenia. *Archives of General Psychiatry* 30:121–128.

Wender, P. H., D. Rosenthal, J. D. Rainer, et al. 1977. Schizophrenic's adopting parents. *Archives of General Psychiatry* 32:777–784.

Wender, P. H., D. Rosenthal, T. P. Zahn, et al. 1971. The psychiatric adjustment of the adopting parents of schizophrenics. *American Journal of Psychiatry* 127:1013–1018.

Wynne, L. C., M. T. Singer, and M. L. Toohey. 1976. Communication of the adoptive parents of schizophrenics. In *Schizophrenia 75,* ed. J. Jorstad and E. Ugelstad. Oslo: Universitat forlaget.

4

A Developmental Theory

THEODORE LIDZ

In this chapter I shall offer a sketch of a theory of schizophrenic disorders that has evolved from studies of the family settings in which schizophrenic patients grew up. Herein Piagetian theories of cognitive development will be fused with psychoanalytic theories of the progressive individuation of the developing person.

The developmental theory I shall outline should not be considered simply as a "family theory" of schizophrenia. It is just as much an existential theory for it holds that the potential for the development of a schizophrenic disorder is inherent in the human condition; if we did not know the syndrome, we would have to search for it as an anticipated aberration of the process of personality development, much as one might search for a potential anomaly of embryonic unfolding. It is also a biological theory, or if you wish, a psychobiological theory, for it rests upon the recognition that the human is integrated at a symbolic level, dependent for adaptation on language and thought, as well as on the realization that the family, even though a social rather than a biological structure, is an essential corollary of man's biological makeup.

The chapter seeks to sketch a comprehensive theory based on observable data, eschewing the positing of potential, though still undetected, genetic and neurochemical factors. It contains ample room for a genetic factor, for which there is rather strong presumptive evidence but still no proof. Such evidence will remain presumptive until it can be determined how the presumed genetic factor or factors affect the organism, as has been the case with various types of mental deficiencies caused by metabolic anomalies.* In any event, almost all who have been convinced that a significant genetic influence exists also recognize that an environmental factor of some sort is also a necessary determinant. I wish to emphasize, however, the importance of a matter that extends far beyond the etiology of schizophrenic disorders. Unless we appreciate that human beings have a dual endowment —a genetic inheritance that they are born with and a cultural heritage that they must assimilate from those who rear and educate them—we can never understand human functioning correctly. It is the neglect of the importance of the family transactions to the child's development or maldevelopment, and of language in human functioning, by so many investigators who are primarily interested in a genetic or neurochemical etiology of schizophrenic disorders to which I object. These are matters that are vital to a viable science of personality development and thereby to the emergence of a scientific psychiatry.

Let me begin by noting several interrelated characteristics of schizophrenic patients. Schizophrenic patients suffer from serious disturbances of thought and communication. This is a matter of definition, for the presence of a thought disorder is the critical, though far from the sole, attribute of that category of psychiatric disorders we term "schizophrenic." Schizophrenic psychoses are those in which symbolic functioning is distorted without degradation of intellectual potential, such as occurs with certain types of brain damage or deterioration or with toxic psychoses.

---

* The incidence of schizophrenia in close relatives, and particularly the concordance of schizophrenia in about twenty to thirty-five percent of monozygotic twins (Tienari 1975; Kringlen 1967; Fischer et al. 1969; Pollin et al. 1966) in contrast to about eight to twelve percent in dizygotic twins makes a genetic factor probable—though the higher rate in same-sexed than opposite-sexed dizygotic twins, particularly female twins, lessens the likelihood. The several adoption studies led by Rosenthal, Kety, and Wender (Kety et al. 1975, see also Chapter 3 of this book; Rosenthal et al. 1974; Wender et al. 1974a; 1974b) as well as the study by Heston (1966) add to the probability but, despite claims of the authors, cannot be considered decisive for a variety of factors. Critiques of these studies have recently been published by Benjamin (1976), Lidz (1976), Kringlen (1976), and Kessler (1976), all of which take exception to the investigators' interpretations of their data.

Those who use the designation "schizophrenia without thought disorder" can be referring only to cases in which there is no gross syntactical or semantic disturbance, and they disregard delusions as evidence of thought disorder; or they are referring to "borderline states" or "pseudoneurotic schizophrenia," which have a psychodynamic relationship to schizophrenic conditions but are not clearly schizophrenic.

Another basic characteristic of schizophrenic patients is their tenuous self boundaries (sometimes termed "ego" boundaries), which lead to confusions between what arises within the self and what outside it and to deficiencies in maintaining the integrity and differentiation of the self. Serious boundary disturbances interfere with the development or maintenance of "object constancy" and thereby inevitably lead to cognitive impairments, as I shall discuss below.

We also now know that the patient's family of origin is always severely disturbed, as demonstrated by our own work (Lidz, Fleck, and Cornelison 1965) and now confirmed by various other investigators. Though it is hazardous to say "always," I know no reason not to do so. Those who disagree with the "always" (Arieti 1974; Bleuler 1976) have not studied the patients' families intensively. Aside from the disturbed and distorting transactions in these families, it has also become clear that one or both parents have markedly disturbed ways of communicating (Bateson et al. 1956; Lidz et al. 1958; Solberg and Blakar 1975; Wynne and Singer 1963a; 1963b; Singer and Wynne 1965a; 1965b; Wynne et al. 1976).

Schizophrenic disorders are failures to achieve or to maintain an integrated personality. For infants to develop into integrated persons, the family—or some planned substitute for it—must nurture them, foster their individuation, provide models for identification, afford a framework for the structuring of their personalities, and provide for their basic socialization and enculturation. Psychoses can also be designated as gross failures of ego functioning, by which I simply mean failures of the capacity to direct the self into the future in a coherent and adaptive manner. Because the capacity to direct the self, as well as to conceptualize a future, depends on symbolic functioning, serious distortions of symbolic functioning can lead to psychosis. All intact infants are born with the capacity to develop symbolic functions, but they must learn their culture's language and ways of thinking as they grow up. As the foundation for gaining this system of meanings and logic is established in the family, distortions of communication within the family can provide a child with a faulty or tenuous foundation in the culture's system of communicating and thinking. Family disturbances, then, if pervasive, can impair both the offspring's symbolic functioning and ability to achieve and maintain a discrete and integrated personality and thereby leave the child vulnerable to becoming schizophrenic. However, the intrafamilial disturbances that lead to an offspring's becoming schizophrenic are specific rather than generalized disorganizations of the family. Our group at Yale (Lidz, Fleck, and Cornelison 1965) has described several such settings, as have others (Wynne et al. 1958; Laing and Esterson 1964). Our findings are too extensive to present here and I shall limit myself to a summary of those which have particular pertinence to my theory.

All of these families had been seriously disturbed and distorted from before the patient was born through the time that the study was being conducted, that is, at least until the patient was an adolescent or young adult. Although some critics hold that the intrafamilial transactions are disturbed at the time of the study because of the difficulties created by the schizophrenic offspring, careful history taking makes such hypotheses extremely unlikely. The problems of individual parents, the problems between parents, and the ways they communicate are deeply engrained in their personalities. In almost every aspect of the family transactions we studied, we found something seriously amiss. In trying to understand our findings, we were forced to move beyond the study of schizophrenic disorders to consider what the family must provide for its offspring in order to foster their proper personality development—their integration as reasonably independent individuals by early adulthood. The scrutiny of these families led us to note influences that have been largely overlooked in developmental psychology, probably because the family is ubiquitous and therefore many of its vital functions for the child have been taken for granted rather than been made the focus of scientific scrutiny.

We found it useful to consider the family's functions in child rearing under four categories.

(1) Parental nurturing, from the total care required by the newborn, through fostering differentiation from the mother while providing the necessary care, affection, and security, to finally promoting the child's separation from the family at the end of adolescence while still offering protection and guidance—functions that are crucial to the child's emotional stability, emotional reactivity and security, and also his cognitive development. In the study of the developmental process of schizophrenic patients, as in the study of the development of autistic children (Mahler 1968), the parents' functions in fostering individuation while providing care, love, security, and guidance come into the limelight.

(2) Structuring the personality. We considered how the dynamic organization of the family channels children's drives and provides a framework around which their personalities gained integration. It seems particularly important for the spouses to form a coalition as parents, maintain the boundaries between the generations, and adhere to their respective gender-linked roles in whatever way these roles are defined in the society. The models for identification and superego development depend not only on the parents as individuals and how each relates to the child but also on the parents' relationship to each other.

(3) Teaching children the basic social roles and institutions of the society and their worth as guides in living and in furnishing motivations. The boundaries of the family cannot be too rigid or impermeable but must enable and even provide interaction with other families and social institutions.

(4) Transmitting the instrumental techniques of the culture, in particular its language, with its system of meanings and logic and its ways of categorizing experiences, but also the culture's mores and ethos.

We now realize that the family in which the schizophrenic patient grows up has failed abysmally to provide these requisites for the child's integrated personality development. This appreciation shifts the focus away from the early mother–infant relationship or, indeed, from any period in the child's life or some specific traumatic occurrence and requires us to take into account the difficulties that existed panphasically throughout the patient's formative years. Whereas frequently the mother was unable to cathect the patient as an infant, this was but one of many problems. The emphasis shifts from trauma, neglect, and causes of fixations to scrutiny of the nature of the transactional field in which these children developed. However, I no longer believe that the appearance of schizophrenia depends on these global disturbances and deficiencies alone but rather on more specific distorting influences that I shall now seek to delineate.

My colleagues and I have tended to divide the families of schizophrenic patients into two types. Soon after our study started, it became obvious that about half of the families were split into two factions because of gross parental conflict; we termed such families *schismatic*. Others were more subtly distorting because the aberrant ways of one parent were accepted as normal by the spouse; these families we termed *skewed*. However, an overlap between these two paradigms occurs rather frequently.

The skewed family pattern is found more often in families with schizophrenic sons than in those with schizophrenic daughters. Here, the striking feature is the so-called "schizophrenogenic" mother, who is extremely intrusive into her child's life but impervious to the child's needs and feelings as a separate individual. However, the father is also important because he is unable to counter his wife's strange ideas of raising children, may not help the child individuate from the mother, and provides his son with a poor model for identification, either by behaving like another child or by being intensely rivalrous with his son for his wife's affection and attention. Although the mother is usually unable to cathect the child as an infant, she soon becomes overprotective and engulfing and is unable to believe the child can survive without her constant supervision. She cannot establish clear boundaries between herself and her son and fails to differentiate her own needs and feelings from his. Feeling incomplete and unfulfilled as a woman, she conveys to her son that her life would be empty and meaningless without him. The boy grows up feeling that it is essential for him to complete his mother's life and that leaving her would be tantamount to killing her. He also feels unable to get along without her, continuing to believe, as he did when a small child, that she is omniscient and omnipotent. He has grandiose expectations of what parental figures can do for him and little faith in his own capacities. His initial identification with his mother is not supplanted by an adequate identification with his father, and the absence of firm boundaries between himself and his mother may lead to fear that closeness can lead to incestuous involvement with his mother, and also to an uncertain, if not a feminine, gender identity. A daughter may remain undifferentiated from the mother, anaclitically needy and with strong homosexual longings. Whatever the father's makeup, he is ineffectual in the home and usually disdained by the mother, who lets her son know that he must grow up to be different from his father to please her and complete her life. In these families the mother's, but sometimes the father's, emotional balance is so precarious that she can retain her equilibrium only by distorting her perception of events to make them coincide with her needs; and she requires other members of the family to distort matters in the same way she does. Because the father does not counter these ways, the family becomes an unreal place into which the child must fit or feel rejected. The child's own feelings and perceptions are invalidated, and the world that the child should come to know, and the value of his or her own emotions as a guide in relating to others, is denied. The child as an adolescent is never confirmed as a separate and competent individual by the parents.

The schismatic pattern more commonly forms the background of female patients. There is overt antagonism between the parents. Each undercuts the worth of the other, and, seeking an ally in the intrafamilial strife, they often compete for the loyalty of the child. The mother, who has little self-esteem and is insecure as a mother, has her self-confidence undermined by the constant derogation of her husband, who has little use for women. Some of the fathers, insecure in their masculinity, sought wives who would docilely cater to their wishes and support their narcissistic needs. The husband takes dissent by his wife as hostile rebelliousness. The mother, usually a poorly organized woman, cannot hold her own against a dominating husband who may be narcissistically grandiose and sometimes paranoidally rigid and suspicious. She conveys a feeling of the meaninglessness or hopelessness of her life. She, too, seeks to be overprotective of her daughter, but the overprotection has a negative, and even an inimical, quality (Alanen 1958). Unhappy in being a woman, she does not gain satisfaction or a sense of completion from a daughter. In these families the fathers are as disturbed as the mothers —often more so because of their paranoid tendencies—but because they are more rigidly organized, they may function rather effectively outside the family. When the father's need for admiration and his unrealistic demands are not met by his wife, he may become seductive toward his daughter in a way that verges on the incestuous, seeking to use her to fill the admiring role his wife is unable or unwilling to occupy. In some cases, though, the father seems pushed into a mothering and rather seductive relationship with the daughter because of the mother's apathy or aversion toward the child. The daughter's developmental process becomes very complicated because in her efforts to gain her father's affection she must seek to become someone very different from her mother. Commonly the child, whether a girl or a boy, is caught in a bind, finding that trying to please one or the other parent provokes rejection and rebuff by the other parent. The child may accept the role of scapegoat and act in a manner that seems to cause the family schism, thus masking the parents' incompatibilities. In so doing, such children sacrifice their own developmental needs to preserve their parents' marriage.

Although the schismatic and skewed configurations may seem very different, they have certain characteristics in common: the use of the child to complete a parent's life or to maintain the parents' marriage, which interferes with the child's development of self-boundaries; the failure of the parent of the same sex as the child to provide an acceptable model for identification, together with the devaluation of this parent by the spouse; the disruptions of the boundaries between the two generations, which leads to incestuous tendencies, faulty oedipal resolutions, and confusions in parental and child functions; the failures of parents to adhere to their respective gender-linked roles; the parents' inability to believe that the child is a separate individual who can increasingly manage on his or her own, and their failure to confirm the child as a competent person; the feelings of emptiness or hopelessness about life conveyed by one or both parents; and the disturbances in verbal and nonverbal communication that pervade the family transactions.

Although disordered intrafamilial communication is an insufficient cause in itself, a child will rarely if ever become schizophrenic unless the intrafamilial communication is markedly disordered (Wynne et al. 1976). My colleagues and I (Lidz et al. 1958) have described how these parents distort their perceptions of experiences to preserve their own tenuous emotional balance and thereby create a strange family setting into which the children must fit themselves or feel rejected. The child's perception of events and feelings is distorted or invalidated to fit the parents' needs and does not properly serve as a guide for relating to persons outside the family. Bateson, Jackson, and their colleagues (1956) first focused attention on how children who become schizophrenic are constantly placed in cognitive as well as emotional double-binds; that is, they are given mutually contradictory messages accompanied by covert threats of rejection if they do not carry out both of the paradoxical messages. They are "damned if they do, and damned if they don't." One common contradictory message that has sweeping consequences occurs when a mother conveys to her son that he must become a great person to be acceptable to her but at the same time he must never become independent of her. In schismatic families the children are caught between the opposing directives of the two parents, and this leads to a split in their inner directives. Wynne and Singer (1963a; 1963b; Singer and Wynne 1965a; 1965b) have drawn attention to the amorphous and fragmented styles of communication of these parents that interfere with the child's ability to maintain the focal attention essential to learn language properly and to communicate coherently. Further, the parents do not let clear concepts stand but create a milieu filled with inconsistencies, contradictory meanings, and the denial of what should be obvious. There are many ways in which the intrafamilial transactions and communication interfere with children's gaining a firm grounding in their culture's system of meanings and logic, confuse their grasp of the world, and leave them despairing about making sense out of events and relationships (Lidz et al. 1958). It has been demonstrated that in some families the disturbed communication has built up over several generations but, of course, it has not been possible to determine how frequently. The familial cognitive disturbances are considered by some (Meehl 1962; McConaghy 1959) to be due to a genetic defect, but this has not been established (Lidz, Wild, et al. 1963; Rosman et al. 1964). And as I shall now develop, there are ample reasons to believe they are fundamentally related to the parents' difficulties in establishing self-boundaries.

Having provided this brief sketch of the family settings and transactions that impede the integrated personality development of offspring who become schizophrenic, I now wish to turn to examine the nature and origins of the schizophrenic thought disorder.* Because the pervasive language and thought disorder, almost always including delusional thinking, distinguishes schizophrenic disorders, it is essential that a theory of schizophrenia explain the nature and origin of this cognitive dysfunction.

The schizophrenic thought disorder has been defined in many ways. Schizophrenic reactions are a type of withdrawal from social interaction, and the thought disorder can be considered as a specifically schizophrenic means of withdrawal by breaking through the confines set by the meanings and logic of the culture. And because the schizophrenic's ways of communicating are idiosyncratic, they in turn increase the patient's isolation. All people are delimited by the meanings and logic of their culture, but without them collaborative interaction with others and relationships beyond infantile dependency are not possible and self-direction is greatly impaired. The schizophrenic patient escapes from irreconcilable conflict, unbearable hopelessness, and loss of self-esteem by breaking through these confines; he finds some living space and pseudodirectives by using his own idiosyncratic meanings and reasoning, but in so doing he impairs his ego functioning and ability to collaborate with others.

When Eugen Bleuler (1911) focused attention on the central

---

* The question of why only one child in a family, or one of two monozygotic twins, becomes schizophrenic is a crucial question, and the intensive studies carried out by the Yale group (Lidz, Fleck, and Cornelison 1965) studied only the families of patients with siblings in order to have an internal control or controls in the form of siblings. The findings that furnish at least a partial answer extend beyond the scope of this essay. They are reported in Lidz, Fleck, et al. 1963.

position of schizophrenic thought disorder, he described it as a derailment of associations. Various investigators have considered the same phenomena as manifestations of deficiencies in forming categories; and I have noted elsewhere how category formation serves as a means of filtering out extraneous associations (Lidz 1968). Norman Cameron's (1938) designation of schizophrenic thinking as "overinclusive" is a highly useful way of describing what happens with the breakdown in categorizing. What has been overlooked is that the overinclusiveness is primarily egocentric, in Piaget's usage of the term. Patients typically believe that what others do or say centers on them, even when it is totally extraneous to them, as in ideas and delusions of reference and persecutory delusional systems; or they believe that their actions, thoughts, or feelings have influence on others and may even be convinced that they magically affect the inanimate universe. Schizophrenic patients, in brief, believe that they are the focal point of events that are in actuality fortuitous or coincidental to their lives. At one pole, paranoid patients perceive that some person or organization of persons is seeking to thwart or injure them; and at the other pole, catatonic patients remain immobile because they believe themselves to be the fulcrum of the universe or because any movement they make can have devastating consequences to the world. Indeed, we are finding evidence that patients become manifestly psychotic when they begin to order their world in such egocentric ways, frantically seeking and finding direction from contingent events (Bowers 1974); and with remission, the egocentric overinclusiveness ceases, or at least diminishes markedly. The schizophrenic is also profoundly egocentric in other ways, as I shall now develop.

We have noted indirectly that the parents of schizophrenic patients, not just the patients themselves, are profoundly egocentric. Many of the characteristics of parents of schizophrenic patients to which I have called attention—their intrusiveness into their child's life but imperviousness to the child's feelings, their inabilities to differentiate their own needs and feelings from their child's or to grasp that the child views situations differently than they do or to believe that the child can manage anything without them, the use of the child to complete their own lives, and so on—have been attributed to the parent's failure to establish proper boundaries between the self and the child. However, such difficulties in forming boundaries are, when viewed from a different orientation, manifestations of a parent's egocentricity—specifically an inability to appreciate that another's feelings and perceptions differ from one's own.

The parent's egocentricity usually differs from the patient's. It is often, though not always, confined to the relationships with family members and particularly to the parent–child relationships, and consists primarily of an inability to recognize that the other person has different feelings, needs, and ways of experiencing than the self. Thus egocentric parents cannot properly accommodate to their children and their needs—an essential characteristic of proper nurturant care—but rather require the immature children to fit themselves to the parents' orientation, to see the world as the parents need to have them see it to help preserve the parents' tenuous equilibrium. In the skewed family the egocentricity of one parent is not countered by the other; in the schismatic family two egocentric parents cannot understand or empathize with one another or the child.

Such patients, having ever needed to adapt themselves to their parents' needs, are alert to the needs and feelings of others and, in contrast to the parents, may be unduly sensitive to them. Thus, the egocentricities of the parent and children are reciprocal in many respects, and whereas they serve to protect the parents' emotional balance, they leave these patients vulnerable because they are directed by parents' needs rather than investing their energies and attention in their own development. Schizophrenic patients come to believe that they cannot manage without their parents and that they can affect their parents profoundly by their own thoughts and feelings. In some respects these patients are more parent-centered than egocentric, but their feelings of being central to their parents' lives lead to feelings of being central and important to everyone, including God, whom the child models as an extension of the parents, as both Freud and Piaget have shown. At the same time they are apt to seek direction from others and readily come to feel controlled by others.

In a sense I have simply been changing the frame of reference of something that many clinicians and investigators have emphasized, namely, that the schizophrenic patient has weak self-boundaries, or in Federn's (1952) terms, fails to cathect ego boundaries and therefore confuses the self and objects, what is internal and external, and what is motivated from within and from without. However, the weak boundaries are not due to an innate defect or to some metabolic abnormality but rather derive from a parent's inability to form boundaries between the self and the patient (Lidz and Lidz 1949). Such deficiencies in boundary formation have widespread ramifications. They prevent the attainment of stable object constancy, impair or prevent proper category formation, confuse gender identity, interfere with superego formation, leave the individual anaclitically dependent, and prevent the attainment of an "ego identity." Here I shall consider primarily the patient's profound egocentricity, which is derived from the parent's egocentricity, in order to clarify the nature of many basic symptoms of schizophrenic disorders, particularly the nature of the cognitive disturbance.

The failure to differentiate clearly between self and nonself, which is so characteristic of schizophrenic patients, is, as Piaget (1926) has described, a normal characteristic of the young child. It represents the egocentricity of the "sensori-motor" period and to some degree the "preoperational" stage of cognitive development. The infant gradually overcomes such egocentricities as he achieves object constancy and differentiates from the mother in the separation–individuation phase that Mahler (1968) has described. Overcoming this initial egocentricity is vital to human development for many reasons but especially for cognitive development because no true category formation can occur unless the self can be excluded from a grouping or category, nor can object constancy be achieved. Developing beyond the oedipal attachment to the mother—recognizing that the mother's life does not center completely on the child—is therefore the final step in overcoming the primary egocentricity. It enables children to enter the stage of "concrete operations," in which they can begin to categorize and at the same time to internalize the maternal object and not need her actual presence to feel secure or to direct their basic behavior.

I have been focusing attention on the relationship of the schizophrenic patients' faulty self-boundaries and the importance of the separation–individuation phase to their development and particularly to their cognitive development, but it is obvious that schizophrenic persons have not remained fixated at this early level of cognitive development. If they had never established boundaries between themselves and their "object" worlds, their language usage and their emotional developments would have been so profoundly affected that they would have become autistic or at least symbiotic psychotic children. Most if not all adult schizophrenics had been able to form concrete categories (or in Piaget's terms, to carry out "concrete operations"), and many could think abstractly (carry out "formal operations"); and some had even shown exceptional capacities for conceptual thinking. However, because of the peculiar family environments in which they had been raised, and because of the irrationalities —including the requirement that they distort their own perceptions in accord with parental needs—their meaning systems, their ways of categorizing experiences, are not firmly based in the culture's system of categorizing. Not only are they more apt to categorize in idiosyncratic ways, perceiving the world less conventionally than others (as do artistically creative persons), but they may also regress into thinking in complexes, or into precategorical, syncretic ways of thinking, particularly when they lose themselves in real or imaginary fusion experiences when seeking intimacy or when they become caught up in some irreconcilable conflict.

In order to understand the cognitive egocentric regressions typical of schizophrenic disorders, we must comprehend the egocentrisms that Piaget (1929) has described in later developmental stages and, insofar as possible, how each type of egocentrism affects object relationships. Piaget has emphasized that children must overcome a different type of egocentricity as they move through each stage of cognitive development. In some respects movement to the subsequent stage of cognitive development means that one has progressed through and overcome to egocentrism of a given stage. Egocentrism, for Piaget, means the overestimation of the power of thought as an instrumental procedure, as well as the distortion of reality to the point of view and the needs of the individual. Both are unconscious, essentially resulting from the failure to distinguish between the subjective and the objective. Egocentrism increases each time that the developmental process brings the child into a new stage of life and concomitantly into a new and untried field of cognitive action, and slowly subsides as the child masters the new field, only to reappear in a new form as the child moves into the next stage of development. Preoperational—or, in the psychoanalytic frame of reference, preoedipal—children must come to differentiate wishes from reality and words from the objects they represent; they must also largely overcome their "animism," their "artificialism" (the belief that all objects are created by men or for men), their "participation" (the belief that their thoughts and actions influence or control nature), and other magical concepts of causality. In particular, preoperational children cannot grasp that events can be fortuitous but rather believe that they always center on them. Such failures to differentiate the subjective and objective—to believe in the efficacy of the wish, to resort to fantasy solutions, to believe in animism, to believe that contingent events center on the self, and so on, are of course very common in schizophrenic patients. The child in the stage of concrete operations (which parallels the so-called latency period) gradually learns that persons in different places do not have the same view of an object that he or she has, and, later, that others may not share his orientation. Children begin to accommodate to the views of others and to overcome the misunderstandings that arise because they do not realize they must orient others to what they are talking about and the distortions that occur because they cannot share the point of view of another or even really grasp that other points of view exist. But while failures to recognize that others perceive and feel differently from the self are common among both schizophrenic patients and their parents, it is the egocentricity that arises early in adolescence that usually has more specific pertinence to the development of schizophrenic states.

It does not seem proper, as has been done so commonly, to place almost all of the emphasis on the events of very early childhood which established the fixation points, the proclivities for regression, the flaws in the personality structure that in turn helped create new problems, and so little emphasis on the later developmental problems which, when not surmounted, create the dam (to follow one of Freud's analogies) that forces the regressive backing up of the developmental flow.

Some schizophrenic patients have never moved completely beyond the stages of preoperational and concrete thinking or beyond anaclitic dependency on a tangible parental object, but many have become capable of more abstract conceptual thinking, have begun to internalize the directives as well as the image of the parental object, have attempted to live on their own, and have then regressed. The first group may be considered as "developmental" (akin to "poor premorbid" or "process") schizophrenics, and the latter group as "regressive (akin to "good premorbid" or "reactive") schizophrenics. However, "developmental" and "regressive" are poles between which most patients are distributed rather than two separate types of schizophrenic disorders.

Schizophrenic patients usually move into mid- or late adolescence before regressing cognitively and emotionally. They reach the developmental period when they are confronted by such psychosocial tasks as achieving independence from the family, a life plan, an ego identity, and a capacity for intimacy—tasks that trouble all adolescents but are particularly difficult if not impossible for those who become schizophrenic because of the intrafamilial impediments to their development, including the limitations of their extrafamilial socialization brought about by the various peculiarities of their parents' beliefs and fears (Lidz, Fleck, and Cornelison 1965). Adolescents also undergo a major transformation that has been disregarded in psychoanalytic developmental theory: cognitively, they enter the stage of formal operations. They now become capable of reflective thinking, of thinking about thinking; and instead of simply proceeding from what is real to what is possible, as they did previously, they can now plan from the possible to the real, and in so doing may become seduced by their capacities to be the master in the mental realm of the possible. The period contains the particular danger that the youth can get lost in mental operations, fantasizing potential futures for himself and the world without becoming involved in the tangible measures required to make them become real, as well as in masturbatory fantasies of sexual gratification rather than overcoming blocks to becoming meaningfully intimate with another person. It is an expansive period of hopes and dreams that, at first, is untempered by the need to prove the feasibility of an ideal or to go through the tangible stages of convincing others and the laborious measures required to bring a plan to realiza- tion. As Inhelder and Piaget (1958) state, "The adolescent goes through a phase in which he attributes an unlimited power to his own thoughts so that the dream of a glorious future or of trans- forming the world through ideas (even if this idealism takes a materialistic form) seems to be not only fantasy but also an effec- tive action which in itself modifies the empirical world. This is obviously a form of cognitive egocentricism" (pp. 345–346). It often takes years for adolescents to overcome the egocentricity that appears with the onset of formal operations, to recognize that one's own ideals and points of view about social issues are never precisely those of others, that thinking things out for oneself is very different from convincing others and from working them out in the real world. It is a characteristic of youth to be carried away by the hypothetical possibilities, to formulate plans mentally and go on to construct imagined brilliant outcomes, but the ability to do so contains a trap into which the vulnerable may fall. Adoles- cents who become schizophrenic overdo their reliance on imagi- nary solutions and gratifications and will even believe they are extraordinary persons with notable attainments because of them and may then paranoidally blame others for not recognizing their worth.

The egocentric aspects of formal operations are overcome through increasing socialization; the youth comes in contact with persons who have different orientations and this forces a reeval- uation of one's own concepts. The process of decentering is aided by "bull sessions," with their endless discussions and ar- guments, by joining and resigning from various social move- ments that are so much a part of youth, but also by undertaking a real job, in which accomplishment rather than imagined results is what counts, and by starting upon a career, which supplies tan- gible directives and role models around which the personality consolidates. The individual's own self-constancy is not shaken by the differing opinions and behavior of others, nor is the other rejected as "bad" simply because his or her views are different.

The first indications that a youth may be in danger of becoming schizophrenic—when his or her future seems to hang in the balance—may come when goals fail to jell and instead become more diffuse and when, rather than moving toward accomplishment, the youth remains in the realm of fantasied achievements and fantasied gratifications. The various grave impediments to personality integration that result from growing up in a disturbed and confusing home now block the development of a coherent gender identity and ego identity and the crucial emergence as an adult; and for some, the difficulties in socializing keep them from overcoming their egocentric overevaluation of their cognitive abilities. When away from the shelter of the family, they feel unbearably lonesome, empty, and rudderless, for they lack the inner structure to replace parental guidance and protection. Often they have not achieved a degree of object constancy that allows them to manage ambivalent feelings about the same person; instead they split the parental object, or are unable to countenance any hostile feelings to a needed parent. When seeking intimacy, fears of being engulfed and losing one's identity cause panic, particularly when in despairing loneliness they regress to fantasies of fusing with a nurturant person. It is, however, not only the inadequacies and distorting influences in the earlier development that create difficulties; they are still caught up in concurrent difficulties with the same disturbed and disturbing parents who raised them. It is not just a matter of infantile and preoedipal fixations that distorted their subsequent developments, though this may be an essential predisposing factor, but the panphasic influences that affected them from birth through adolescence and the continuing confusing current relationships with their most significant persons that interfere with forward movement, lead to despair and sometimes to terror, and initiate regression. Persons who become schizophrenic, however, have in some significant way never achieved adult object constancy— not simply the internalization of images of significant objects in the object's absence but the making part of themselves the parental directives, affection, and presence more or less abstracted from the parent's image. Of course, the onset of a schizophrenic disorder often comes later than adolescence or early adulthood, but in many such instances the patients had not actually mastered the essential tasks of adolescence, and if no longer caught up in problems with their families of origin, they have simply transferred them to those who had become the significant persons in their lives; and in others, a relationship that permitted them to maintain a precarious balance for some years had been lost or undermined.

As part of their inability to move through adolescence, youths who become schizophrenic fail to decenter cognitively. Feeling hopeless about the future and despairing of ever becoming a person in their own right, such youths develop more elaborate fantasy solutions and regress cognitively as well as emotionally. Poorly grounded in reality testing, and with tenuous boundaries between the self and others, they seek ways out of their real developmental dilemmas by falling back to childhood forms of egocentric cognition, as well as by seeking security through fusion with another. All egocentrism, whatever the specific type and from whatever stage of development, is bound together by the common characteristic of reliance on the omnipotence of thought. The schizophrenic can again give precedence to wish over reality, to belief in parental omnipotence and the magic of the wish. Desperately seeking meaning, for an answer to the why and how of living that schizophrenics feel is hidden from them but known to others, and for direction into the future, everything takes on heightened relevance and becomes personally meaningful. They find that every fortuitous occurrence applies to them, as they again believe themselves central to all that happens. To some degree they will regress even more profoundly and, like the early preoedipal child, confuse the self and nonself and what arises within the self and what comes from outside of the self. The results are far-reaching and devastating. There is an accompanying regression in the level of object constancy that can reach back to considering the same person to be a different individual when satisfying than when unsatisfying, to believing in the omnipotence of parental figures, and so on. The categorizations developed are now seriously impaired; and with the filtering function of categories lost, inappropriate associations intrude and derail thought and communication. When the onset is acute, the process is augmented by anxiety and panic, for with stimulation of the sympathetic nervous system and an outpouring of epinephrine, the physiologic filtering of input by the reticular activating system is lowered. According to the individual and the situation, thinking becomes preconceptual, or even syncretic and metonymic, permitting the patient to connect anything that is spatially or temporally contiguous and thus further justify egocentric distortions.

The breakdown of proper category formation has another potential consequence (Lidz 1968). Various authorities have noted that the formation of boundaries between the self and nonself is basic to all category formation. Since experience is continuous and categories are discrete, boundaries must be placed between categories by repressing what lies between them, starting with what is self and what is not self and what is inside and what is outside the self—the fusions between child and mother such as nursing at the breast, and fantasies of fusion in sexual relations, as well as taboos on excretions and secretions that were part of the self but become nonself (Leach 1966). We may also posit a similar fundamental need to place taboos upon, or repress, whatever might confuse the categories of parent and child and of male and female. These are precisely the areas in which parents of schizophrenics are apt to fail to foster essential repression. With the regression to childhood types of egocentric thinking and the disruption of categorical thinking, persons in whom the boundaries between these basic differentiations had never been firmly established may become particularly vulnerable to preoccupation with material that lies between categories—with an intercategorical realm concerned with fusions of the self and mother, with polymorphous perverse fantasies concerning orifices and genitals, with cannibalistic impulses, with dreamlike notions of being of the opposite sex, and other such material that is normally eliminated from awareness as a child grows up—material that can have little conscious representation and for which no clear-cut categories exist. It is in this intercategorical realm that some schizophrenic patients spend much of their time: a world which we, as therapists, have grave difficulty penetrating and about which we have but fragmentary glimpses but which erupts into the patient's talk and associations as from another world. It is not just the eruption of an internalized version of reality that is somewhat akin to our own, but more of a nether world, a world that is antipodal, composed of what we have learned to keep out of most of our fantasies and to some extent even out of our dreams.* Still, no matter how profound the regression, schizophrenic patients are not infants nor even children, and much of what they had acquired cognitively remains available to them and limits the extent of the cognitive disorder. Further, what they had acquired is not, or need not be, permanently lost.

The escape through the abandonment of the culture's system of meanings and logic is not a way open to all but only to those whose boundaries remain tenuous and whose foundations in the culture's ways of thinking and reality testing are faulty. While this escape may seem tempting, it is profoundly isolating and often filled with terror of punishment by extrojected and hallucinated superego figures; therefore patients frequently struggle to escape, and not all persons who become schizophrenic remain so. However, the condition can readily consolidate as delusional insights expand to explain the perplexing world in which the patient was raised and lives, to clarify the reasons for failure, to enable the continuation of some gratification through retreat into fantasy, and particularly to defend against the panic that often comes when boundaries vanish and leave the individual prey to threatening intrusions or loss of self. It can continue because schizophrenic patients no longer test the validity of their ideas by their instrumental utility or by how they foster collaboration with others (Lidz et al. 1958).

I have not sought to account for the entire range of schizophrenic thought disorders. Paranoid delusions and hallucinations are also concerned with boundary problems and egocentric cognition, in which patients project their own feelings and impulsions onto others and may also project parental introjects or edicts as a means of controlling their own dangerous impulses. When the situation is no longer acute, the schizophrenic usually can think competently except in areas that confuse or create emotional turmoil. Although some schizophrenics have never

---

* Though clearly related, I do not think this intercategorical realm is synonymous with primary process thinking. Indeed, the division of thought into conscious, preconscious, and unconscious, or into primary and secondary process thinking, is limiting. Certain types of "primitive" thinking have the characteristics of Piaget's preoperational thought rather than Freud's primary process, which Freud modeled after dreamwork.

reached the stage of formal operations, others have; the question is not whether such schizophrenics are capable of conceptual thinking but rather under what circumstances the ability to categorize breaks down or what leads to egocentric cognitive regression as well as libidinal regression. In chronic patients we find still other types of thought disorders, such as evasive ambiguity, constricting literality (Lorenz 1963), reversal of intent, and so on as a defense against ever again becoming involved in a meaningful relationship, or against experiencing unbearable despair, and these techniques of defense may overshadow all other cognitive distortions.

I believe that this sketch of a theory of schizophrenic disorders brings coherence to the basic phenomenology of the syndrome and clarifies their origins by utilizing the findings of family studies about the patient's developmental settings and difficulties. The theory focuses attention on the vulnerability of the adolescent to disorganization and regression because adolescence is the time when personality integration must jell, but also because the cognitive egocentricity that comes with the start of conceptual thinking opens the way for the adolescent to leave reality and fall back on fantasy solutions. The theory also notes how persons who become schizophrenic are particularly vulnerable because the family settings in which they grew up failed to provide the requisites for the integrated development of the child, and specifically because parental egocentricity interfered with boundary formation between parent and child and distorted the intrafamilial communication. Unable to surmount the developmental tasks of adolescence and lacking inner structure, the schizophrenic patient regresses to earlier egocentric, overinclusive types of thinking as well as withdrawing and regressing emotionally.

DISCUSSION

Your position is that a family disturbance is always involved in schizophrenic illness. Would you comment on atypical family situations, such as one-parent families, or families in other cultures?

I believe that schizophrenic patients always come from disturbed or distorting family settings. We asked colleagues in New York and Boston as well as New Haven to send us schizophrenic patients who, they believed, came from stable families. We studied three or four such families closely, and it became apparent that they were seriously disturbed, though the difficulties were not apparent to someone outside the family. We excluded one-parent families from our intensive study, but in an earlier study Dr. Ruth Lidz and I (1949) found that about forty percent of upper-middle-class schizophrenics came from homes broken by divorce, permanent separation of the parents, or the death of a parent. I cannot say much about parents in very divergent cultures, but studies in Japan, Finland, Germany, Israel, and Tunisia have come up with very similar findings. I understand that Dr. David Rosenthal has been studying the incidence of schizophrenia in persons raised in kibbutzim, but I do not know the results. Drs. Wynne and Singer found that parents of schizophrenics in Lebanon and Japan showed the same communicative difficulties as those in the United States.

Some excellent clinicians, including Silvano Arieti and Manfred Bleuler, believe that not all or even most schizophrenic patients grew up in such families, but they have not studied the families carefully. It should be noted that Ernst (1956) checked the records at the Burgholzli Hospital and found that most of their schizophrenics had come from disturbed families; when he examined the remainder personally, he found that they too had the same problems. I do not know why Manfred Bleuler has not accepted Ernst's findings.

Do you think there are some consistent intrapsychic problems in parents of schizophrenic persons?

I believe that one or both suffer from difficulties in maintaining boundaries between the self and the patient, and often between the self and others—at least other family members. They are egocentric in ways I have described. We must recognize that serious boundary problems have far-reaching intrapsychic effects—lack of object constancy, improper concept formation, and other basic ego defects as well as deficiencies in superego formation.

Are "boundary problems" the same as psychopathology?

I would say that boundary problems *are* psychopathology and that we are entering a phase in the study of psychopathology in which the focus will be on the course of the separation–individuation process, its aberrations, and how various deficiencies in the process lead to different types of psychopathology.

I wish to add that children who have one parent with fairly serious boundary problems are not always seriously affected. The other parent may compensate; substitute figures may be important; and a mother with a boundary problem may offset the difficulty by warmth and the like. Sometimes parents are so obviously disturbed that children discount their communications and behavior.

In light of what you have said, would you comment on treating a schizo-phrenic person individually or within the family?

If the question is whether schizophrenic patients should be treated in individual therapy or conjoint family therapy, I would say preferably both. Although some believe that conjoint family therapy is the preferred means of treatment for schizophrenic patients, this has not been my experience. Family therapy can help and is often essential, for it enables the patient to gain a new perspective of the parents and family transactions; it can help release the patient from accepting the parents' ways of thinking and feeling as his own, and so on. It can also provide support for the parents, as well as help them change their attitudes. However, these families do not change easily, and helping the patient achieve independence may be the only beneficial outcome of the family therapy. Further, not all family therapy need be conjoint therapy. There are times when working with the parents singly or as a couple can be more effective. In general, however, I believe individual therapy is also necessary. The results of the years of noxious family transactions have been internalized and are not likely to be undone simply by changing the current situation.

Would you give us your ideas on "genetic loading" in schizophrenia?

I think it probable that there is some genetic loading, but up to now it has not been proven. It is presumptive, and much is gained by challenging presumptions. A careful examination of Dr. Kety's data will show that the major difference between the biological relatives of schizophrenics and of control adoptees is found in the patient's half-siblings. Kringlen (1976), as I, believes that this can indicate an environmental influence—and certainly half-siblings cannot be used statistically in the same manner as first-degree relatives. The heavy reliance on diagnoses of "latent" and "probable latent" schizophrenia to achieve significant results is also disturbing to some of us. One more item in Dr. Rosenthal's studies of the adopted-away offspring of schizophrenics: if we limit ourselves to the offspring of so-called "process schizophrenics," we find that only one out of thirty had become definitely schizophrenic; and yet it has always been considered that it would be the offspring of the so-called "true" or "process" schizophrenics who would be affected genetically and have a high incidence of schizophrenia.

REFERENCES

Alanen, Y. O. 1958. The mothers of schizophrenic patients. *Acta Psychologica et Neurologica Scandinavica* (supplement) 124.

Arieti, S. 1974. An overview of schizophrenia from a predominantly psychological approach. *American Journal of Psychiatry* 121:241–249.

Bateson, G., D. Jackson, et al. 1956. Toward a theory of schizophrenia. *Behavioral Science* 1:251–264.

Benjamin, L. S. 1976. A reconsideration of the Kety and associates study of genetic factors in the transmission of schizophrenia. *American Journal of Psychiatry* 133:1129–1133.

Bleuler, E. 1911. *Dementia praecox or the group of schizophrenias.* New York: International Universities Press, 1950.

Bleuler, M. 1976. The long-term course of the schizophrenic psychoses. In *Annual review of the schizophrenic syndrome,* vol 6, 1976, ed. R. Cancro. New York: Brunner/Mazel.

Bowers, M. 1974. *Retreat from sanity.* New York: Human Sciences Press.

Cameron, N. 1938. *Reasoning, regression and communication in schizophrenics.* Columbus: Psychological Review Co.

Ernst, K. 1956. Geordnete Familienverhältnisse späterer Schizophrener im Lichte einer Nachuntersuchung. *Archiv fur Psychiatrie und Nervenkrankheiten vereinigt mit Zeitschrift fur die Gesamte Neurologie und Psychiatrie* 194:355–357.

Federn, P. 1952. *Ego psychology and the psychoses,* ed. E. Weiss. New York: Basic Books.

Fischer, M., B. Harvald, et al. 1969. A Danish twin study of schizophrenia. *British Journal of Psychiatry* 115:981–990.

Heston, L. 1966. Psychiatric disorders in foster home reared children of schizophrenic mothers. *British Journal of Psychiatry* 112:819–825.

Inhelder, B., and J. Piaget. 1958. *The growth of logical thinking from childhood to adolescence.* New York: Basic Books.

Kessler, S. 1976. Progress and regress in the research on the genetics of schizophrenia. *Schizophrenia Bulletin* 2:434–439.

Kety, S., D. Rosenthal, et al. 1975. Mental illness in the biological and adoptive families of adopted individuals who have become schizophrenic: a preliminary report based on psychiatric interviews. In *Genetic research in psychiatry,* ed. R. Fieve, D. Rosenthal, and H. Brill. Baltimore: Johns Hopkins University Press.

Kringlen, E. 1967. *Heredity and environment in the functional psychoses.* Oslo: Universitatsforlaget.

_____. 1976. Twins—still our best method. *Schizophrenia Bulletin* 2:429–433.

Laing, R., and A. Esterson. 1964. *Sanity, madness and the family.* London: Tavistock Publications.

Leach, E. 1966. Anthropological aspects of language: animal categories and verbal abuse. In *New directions in the study of language,* ed. E. Lenneberg. Cambridge: MIT Press.

Lidz, R. W., and T. Lidz. 1949. The family environment of schizophrenic patients. *American Journal of Psychiatry* 106:332–345.

Lidz, T. 1968. The family, language, and the transmission of schizophrenia. In *The transmission of schizophrenia,* ed. D. Rosenthal and S. Kety. Oxford: Pergamon Press.

_____. 1976. Commentary on "A critical review of recent adoption, twin, and family studies of schizophrenia: behavioral genetics perspectives" by I. Gottesman and J. Shields. *Schizophrenia Bulletin* 2:402–412.

Lidz, T., A. Cornelison, et al. 1958. Intrafamilial environment of the schizophrenic patient, part 6: The transmission of irrationality. *A.M.A. Archives of Neurology and Psychiatry* 79:305–316.

Lidz, T., S. Fleck, and A. Cornelison. 1965. *Schizophrenia and the family*. New York: International Universities Press.

Lidz, T., S. Fleck, et al. 1963. Schizophrenic patients and their siblings. *Psychiatry* 26:1–18.

Lidz, T., C. Wild, et al. 1963. Thought disorders in the parents of schizophrenic patients: a study utilizing the Object Sorting Test. *Journal of Psychiatric Research* 1:193–200.

Lorenz, M. 1963. Criticism as approach to schizophrenic language. *Archives of General Psychiatry* 9:235–245.

Mahler, M. 1968. *On human symbiosis and the vicissitudes of individuation*. New York: International Universities Press.

McConaghy, N. 1959. The use of an object sorting test in elucidating the hereditary factor in schizophrenia. *Journal of Neurology, Neurosurgery and Psychiatry* 22:243–245.

Meehl, P. 1962, Schizotaxia, schizotypy, schizophrenia. *American Psychologist* 17:827–838.

Piaget, J. 1926. *The language and thought of the child*. New York: Harcourt, Brace, Jovanovich.

_____. 1929. *The child's conception of the world*. Paterson: Littlefield, Adams, 1963.

Pollin, W., J. Stabenau, et al. 1966. Life history differences in identical twins discordant for schizophrenia. *American Journal of Orthopsychiatry* 36:492–509.

Rosenthal, D., P. Wender, et al. 1973. The adopted-away offspring of schizophrenics. In *Annual review of the schizophrenic syndrome*, vol. 3, 1973, ed. R. Cancro. New York: Bruner/Mazel.

Rosman, B., C. Wild, et al. 1964. Thought disorders in the parents of schizophrenic patients: a further study utilizing the Object Sorting Test. *Journal of Psychiatric Research* 2:211–221.

Singer, M., and L. C. Wynne. 1965a. Thought disorder and family relations of schizophrenics, part 3: Methodology using projective techniques. *Archives of General Psychiatry* 12:187–200.

_____. 1965b. Thought disorder and family relations of schizophrenics, part 4: Results and implications. *Archives of General Psychiatry* 12:201–212.

Solberg, H., and R. Blakar. In press. Communication efficiency in couples with and without a schizophrenic offspring.

Tienari, P. 1975. Schizophrenia in Finnish male twins. In *Studies of schizophrenia*, ed. M. H. Laker. *British Journal of Psychiatry*, special publication no. 10. Ashford, England: Headley Brothers.

Wender, P., D. Rosenthal, et al. 1974a. Crossfostering: a research strategy for clarifying the role of genetic and experiental factors in the etiology of schizophrenia. *Archives of General Psychiatry* 30:121–128.

———. 1974b. The psychiatric adjustment of the adopting parents of schizophrenics. *American Journal of Psychiatry* 127:1013–1018.

Wynne, L. C., I. Ryckoff, et al. 1958. Pseudo-mutuality in the family relations of schizophrenics. *Psychiatry* 21:205–220.

Wynne, L. C., and M. Singer. 1963a. Thought disorder and family relations of schizophrenics, part 1: A research strategy. *Archives of General Psychiatry* 9:191–198.

———. 1963b. Thought disorder and family relations of schizophrenics, part 2: A classification of forms of thinking. *Archives of General Psychiatry* 9:199–206.

Wynne, L. C., M. Singer, and M. L. Toohey. 1976. Communication of the adoptive parents of schizophrenics. In *Schizophrenia 75*, ed. J. Jorstad and E. Ugelstad. Oslo: Universitatforlaget.

PART THREE

Bioscientific Research and Treatment

5

The Evolution of a Scientific Nosology

GERALD L. KLERMAN

The concept of disease is not a given. It must be achieved as a result of the accumulation of research. The criteria for considering a state a disease developed in the seventeenth century in the writings of Thomas Sydenham and others, who conceived of a disease as having characteristic symptoms and a natural history. For general medicine the disease concept was crystallized in the mid-nineteenth century by Rudolf Virchow, who united Sydenham's observation of clinical patterns with the findings of Pasteur and others. It was not until the late nineteenth century that this concept of disease as being defined by etiology was applied to mental disorders by the generation of Emil Kraepelin and Eugen Bleuler. Although "schizophrenia" was not Kraepelin's term, it was he who synthesized the clinical observations of a number of continental European psychiatrists, mostly German but also French, from about 1820 to 1895.

Kraepelin was born in 1859, the same year as Sigmund Freud. Yet in conventional thinking Freud is regarded as part of the modern era and Kraepelin is seen as belonging to an older era. Kraepelin's achievements are mainly embodied in his textbook, which went through eight editions. His textbook was significant in the history of psychiatry not because it was the first textbook of psychiatry but because it was one of the first to approach mental illness in terms of causation and etiology, using the principles of modern scientific medicine.

Today, we have been so influenced by modern medicine that

we take for granted that the classification of diseases should be based on the principle of causation. We forget that at the beginning of the nineteenth century the few textbooks of medicine that existed did not embody the principle of causation. This principle was a product of morbid pathology from autopsy findings and of the discoveries of bacteriology later in the century.

After classifying as many cases of mental illness as possible by etiology—those due to infection, to endocrine disorders, and so on—Kraepelin was left with a large group of patients whose psychoses began in young adulthood and went on for many years but who had relatively few deaths, in contrast to patients with psychoses associated with infectious diseases. Among those in this last category who died, the usual techniques of staining or gross dissection at autopsy revealed no cause of death. Kraepelin proposed that these psychotic conditions with no established etiology be further divided into two groups, which he called "dementia praecox" and "manic-depressive insanity." He justified this division on the basis of clinical features during the acute illness, long term course, and outcome.

According to Kraepelin's description, manic-depressive insanity is characterized by strong affects, either depressed or elated, in the presence of clear intellectual function; patients with these features improved from their acute episodes without intellectual impairment but were likely to have multiple recurrences. This description involved the union of the presenting symptoms with the course. Similarly, dementia praecox was described as beginning in young adulthood and ultimately resulting in impairment of intellectual functioning as its end stage—in other words, a dementia. Kraepelin observed that the presenting symptoms of these patients also were a flattening of affect and a "loss of will." He united these two clinical features, presentation and outcome, with a presumed etiology, which he at various times stated was hereditary or was due to metabolic features. Considerable debate has ensued over the defining criteria of schizophrenia— whether they are the presenting clinical symptoms or the outcome. At the current time most neo-Kraepelinians resolve this dilemma by splitting the schizophrenic diagnosis into these two criteria.

As is apparent from his textbooks of psychiatry, Eugen Bleuler in many respects was in the same tradition as Kraepelin. However, Bleuler disagreed with Kraepelin's theory that cognitive intellectual impairments were a dementia. Bleuler proposed the term "organic brain syndrome" for those disorders of brain function which manifest themselves by confusion, loss of memory, and fluctuation in orientation to time, place, and person. He noted that these types of dysfunctions were not present in the patients with dementia praecox, whose defect in cognition was rather from difficulties in association. Since his theoretical point of view was from associational psychology and he explicitly applied Freud's psychoanalytic ideas which made use of associational concepts, he attempted to explain the defect in the thinking of these patients as a failure in normal processes of association rather than as a manifestation of dementia, as originally proposed by Kraepelin. When Bleuler wrote his monograph on schizophrenia, his associates at the Burgholzi Hospital included Jung and Abraham; and in these early writings (which he seemed later to retract) Bleuler put forth his own hope that Freud's theory of associations would be a sufficient explanation for the deficiencies of schizophrenics.

In his later years Bleuler grew more pessimistic about a psychogenic cause of schizophrenia. He encouraged the work of his associates, particularly Jung, to understand the content of the patient's behavior in terms of the patient's private meanings. Bleuler created the term "autism" for the highly personal associational chain of meanings of schizophrenics— meanings that were understandable only in terms of the developmental history of the individual.

Bleuler also differed from Kraepelin with regard to the nature of the disturbance of affect. Kraepelin had characterized patients with dementia praecox as having flat affect. Bleuler noted that in addition there was ambivalence, that is, the simultaneous appearance of opposing affects. Today there is a concensus among clinical and theoretical approaches that the affective disturbances in schizophrenia first described by Kraepelin are the end stage of the chronic process. In the early stages multiple affective states—anger, sadness, depression, anxiety—are present in intense degrees and are often highly fluctuating. Prior to World War II, however, there were heated debates as to whether or not

the presence of affect ruled out the diagnosis of dementia praecox or schizophrenia.

Bleuler's term "schizophrenia" did not imply split personality
which is the common but incorrect definition of the term in popular literature today. He used it within his associational theory of
psychology to emphasize the dissociation within the stream of
consciousness, the loss of associational meaning, the split of affect from ideation, and the loss of integrated functioning of the
personality. Diagnostically, he used the term quite incon-
sistently, as implied in the title of his monograph, *Dementia
Praecox or the Group of Schizophrenias.* One meaning of
"schizophrenia" was that it was a symptom of a disorder with
multiple etiologies, hence, a group of disorders. At times he
seems to speak of psychogenic causation but at other times of hereditary etiology. He was also inconsistent as to outcome. In the
follow-up statistics of his own institution, the Burgholzi Hospital, about a thirty-percent recovery rate is reported; yet he stated
elsewhere that the disorder never allows complete restitution.
So he seemed to be inconsistent in his writings both as to
whether he himself would accept a psychogenic etiology and as
to whether he held to an inevitable poor outcome for the disorder.

Thus, for the generation of whom Kraepelin and Bleuler were
the leading spokesmen, the most pressing clinical problem was
the development of criteria for separating the large group of psychotic conditions into groups based on available evidence of causation. Kraepelin's main achievement was twofold: first, he was
the most persistent in applying the etiological approach to mental disorders, in contrast to the predominantly symptomatic approaches that prevailed during the earlier part of the nineteenth
century; and second, he delineated two main types of psychoses
—dementia praecox and manic-depressive insanity—from
among those of the group without any apparent etiology. Bleuler
later renamed dementia praecox "schizophrenia" because of his
observation that the cognitive disturbance was not that of dementia but was that of an associational defect.

The period subsequent to Bleuler, from about 1910–1950, was
marked by theoretical acrimony and limited therapeutic success,
although most psychiatrists in both Europe and North American

quickly accepted Bleuler's criteria for defining the syndrome. Many unsuccessful attempts were made to find biological causes via searches for anatomical defects in the brain or various toxins elsewhere in the body fluids. The record of therapeutic efforts was perhaps dismal. The group of people labeled schizophrenic during this period were unfortunately subjected to many horrendous interventions in the name of treatment. When theories of generalized infection were in vogue, all the teeth of schizophrenics were removed. When the theory of autointoxication was popular in the 1920s, the high colonic enema was all the rage, and that sometimes meant total colonic resection for schizophrenics. Other theories led to castration or sterilization. There is hardly an organ of the body that was not excised in the name of therapy.

By World War II the biological approach had fallen into disrepute. This adventure in psychiatry had reached its height in 1911 with the discovery of the spirochete as the cause of general paresis. It was hoped that this advance would soon be followed by a similar discovery in the large group of so-called functional psychoses, schizophrenia or manic-depressive insanity. But for these disorders the efforts using available biological techniques were failures. Not only did cures not materialize, but just getting out of the hospital was an achievement if not a miracle. Eighty percent of patients admitted to public mental hospitals were never discharged.

In the 1950s two developments occurred almost simultaneously that revolutionized the treatment of schizophrenia. The first was the development of rauwolfia and the phenothiazines, the earliest of the so-called tranquilizers. These drugs provided effective treatments for the acute symptomatic manifestations of many schizophrenic psychoses. They also helped shorten the stay of patients in institutions and increased the percentage of patients discharged. The second development was a new psychosocial approach to the hospital milieu and a new set of attitudes toward the treatment of schizophrenics. A number of novel policies were introduced, first in Britain and then in the United States, including an "open door" policy, the avoidance of seclusion and restraint, the development of large group techniques such as therapeutic communities, the upgrading of the status and training of nonprofessionals, a conscious effort to bring about early discharge, attempts to break down administrative and other barriers between the hospital and the community, and the involvement of the family. This series of developments became known as social psychiatry. It is unfortunate, in a sense, that these two major developments—neuroleptic drugs and social psychiatry—occurred at the same time, because each has obscured the relative contribution of the other to the reduction of the number of patients in mental hospitals and to the improved outlook for the acute schizophrenic process.

The Neo-Kraepelinians

American, British, and Canadian psychiatry is today in the midst of a Kraepelinian revival that is becoming the dominant force among research and academic leaders (Klerman 1977a). In contrast, the Meyerian school (named after Adolf Meyer, 1866–1950) is currently in a phase of decline in American psychiatry. The Meyerian approach stresses the importance of personal experience and the uniqueness of the individual in his social context, in contrast to the Kraepelinian emphasis on categorizing diseases, an emphasis derived from continental European medicine (Klerman 1976).

The neo-Kraepelinian credo includes nine propositions:

(1) Psychiatry is a branch of medicine.
(2) Psychiatry should utilize modern scientific methodologies and base its practice on scientific knowledge.
(3) Psychiatry treats people who are sick and who require treatment for mental illnesses.
(4) There is a boundary between the normal and the sick.
(5) There are discrete mental illnesses. Mental illnesses are not myths. There is not one but many mental illnesses. It is the task of scientific psychiatry, as of other medical specialties, to investigate the causes, diagnosis, and treatment of these mental illnesses.
(6) The focus of psychiatric physicians should be particularly on the biological aspects of mental illness.
(7) There should be an explicit and intentional concern with diagnosis and classification.

(8) Diagnostic criteria should be codified, and a legitimate and valued area of research should be to validate such criteria by various techniques. Further, departments of psychiatry in medical schools should teach these criteria and not depreciate them, as has been the case for many years.

(9) In research efforts directed at improving the reliability and validity of diagnosis and classification, statistical techniques should be utilized.

Who are the proponents of this point of view? The initial statement of the neo-Kraepelinians was the textbook of Meyer-Gross, Slader, and Roth, originally published in Britain in 1951. The book was a resounding and aggressive affirmation of the Kraepelinian approach, criticizing psychoanalysis, psychotherapy, and social psychiatry. In this country the neo-Kraepelinian point of view has been most strongly identified with the group at Washington University in St. Louis, whose leading spokesman are Eli Robins (1977), Sam Guze (1970), and George Winokur (Winokur et al. 1969). Recently, they have been joined by a New York contingent including Donald Klein (Klein and Davis 1969), whose book on diagnosis and drug treatment has probably been the most influential textbook of psychopharmacology in this country. Klein has repeatedly asserted that psychiatrists cannot prescribe drug treatment appropriately without a careful description of the patient's symptoms and syndromes. Another New York investigator identified with the neo-Kraepelinian approach is Robert Spitzer (Spitzer and Wilson 1968), chairperson of the American Psychiatric Association Task Force that is drafting the third edition of the *Diagnostic and Statistical Manual*. The first draft of this volume has been met with controversy over the strongly descriptive approach it takes to psychopathology.

The Kraepelinian revival is part of the general movement of psychiatry towards greater integration with medicine. This movement has multiple sources, professional, economic, social, scientific. Whatever its sources, the consequence for psychiatry is a greater concern for medical identity. Applied to schizophrenia, there is greater attention to diagnosis in the classical medical tradition and to biological causes and treatments of this disorder. To better understand these developments requires exploration of the "medical model."

The Medical Model

The medical model has become a code word for controversy and debate, a slogan with which to rally one's allies or to castigate one's enemies. To psychiatrists concerned about defending their health insurance prerogatives, the medical model is an umbrella to justify continued support from Blue Cross, Blue Shield, or Aetna. To psychologists and other nonmedical practitioners anxious to be included under health insurance, the medical model refers to a narrow biological approach to the treatment of psychological problem. To behavior therapists, who apply the methods of B. F. Skinner, the medical model applies to dynamic psychotherapy and psychoanalysis, which they attack for postulating "underlying conflicts" of which symptoms are only manifest behaviors. (It is ironic that this extension of the medical model to psychoanalysis would be rejected by a substantial group of nonpsychiatric physicians.) To black militants in an urban ghetto, the medical model is a term of contempt for the futile attempt of the community mental health center to treat social ills by treating individuals, whom the militants regard as victims rather than patients.

The medical model is being widely criticized within medicine and within other professions, but it is also often misunderstood. As I understand it, the medical model includes at least three components. They are:

(1) *The disease concept.* This is a theory of illness that evolved in the eighteenth century and is now held throughout Western industrial civilization.

(2) *The sick role.* As sociologists such as Parsons (1951) and Fox (1968) and anthropologists such as Fabraga (Fabraga et al. 1968) have pointed out, every known society has a category of the "sick role" for a special class of deviance, even non-Western societies that do not have modern notions of biology such as bacteriology or catecholamines. The sick role carries with it a set of rights and prerogatives, and mechanisms are specified whereby this role can legitimately be conferred on certain individuals by another group within society, the "healers."

(3) *The health care system.* As society becomes more specialized and differentiated, the roles of both the sick and the healer become more complex. In modern industrial society there is a complex health care system that includes various kinds of specialists among healers, such as nurses, doctors, technicians, as well as complex institutions such as hospitals and universities and, recently, fiscal mechanisms such as health insurance and Social Security. In part, the debate over whether or not schizophrenia or anxiety are "diseases" is a conflict over whether individuals exhibiting such behaviors are legitimately to be given the rights and prerogatives of the sick role and whether or not the complex and powerful apparatus of the health care system shall serve their needs. While most of the discussion in the literature is on the nature and theory of disease, implicit in the debates are practical decisions as to who shall be considered sick, who shall be treated within the medical system, and under what fiscal auspices.

Looked at in these terms, mental illness and the medical model are social constructs; they are inventions of modern society that attempt to make sense of and deal with the real phenomena of pain, distress, anguish, and disability experienced by certain individuals. However, to say that the medical model or the concept of mental illness is a social construct is not to say that it is a myth or that it is invalid. All social constructs are not myths and they are not necessarily untrue. After all, "the rights of man," the electron, and the university are also social constructs. They are not facts given in nature, but rather are complex ideas developed by historical forces and legitimated by consent. The concept of illness is not arbitrary but reflects areas of shared consensus, embodying truths arrived at by rules of evidence.

The application of the medical model to mental illness was an achievement of the nineteenth century, when Philippe Pinel at the Salpêtrière was responsible for bringing medical leadership to the asylums. For centuries Western Europe had had institutions for lunatics, but these asylums had not been considered appropriate for medical supervision. Usually they were run by religious orders or were parts of jails or prisons. Furthermore, the courts had not distinguished "madness" and "badness" as clearly as became the norm in the early part of the nineteenth century, as a result of the eighteenth century Enlightenment. This distinction between being mad and being bad was regarded as a major humanitarian gain, motivated by humane and benevolent intents.

Modern critics of psychiatry as a medical specialty and of schizophrenia as a mental illness would now have social policy rule that the humanitarian achievements of the Enlightenment were, by some twist of logic and history, an act of tyranny and of self-seeking by psychiatrists. Among these critics are two groups of special relevance to any discussion of the concept of schizophrenia: the "antipsychiatrists" and the "labeling theorists."

The antipsychiatrists are, interestingly enough, psychiatrists who criticize the medical basis of psychiatric practice. They are deeply concerned about the extent to which the mental health field is part of the health system. Their most prominent spokesmen are Thomas Szasz (1961) in the United States, and R. D. Laing (1967) in Great Britain. While there have been many psychiatric critics of specific theories or therapies within psychiatry, the antipsychiatrists pose the radical issue as to the very basis for psychiatry's being a part of medicine. In their criticism of diagnosis and drug therapy they challenge the application of the medical model to mental illness in general and schizophrenia in particular. They question the claim that drugs, psychotherapy, or any other behavioral intervention is in fact therapeutic for schizophrenic persons. Their challenge is also moral and political—they hold that in the guise of therapy, potent methods of behavior control are being used for social control rather than for the best interest of the individual schizophrenic patient.

Closely allied to the antipsychiatrists are the "labeling theorists" from sociology. Sociologists such as Scheff (1964) and social psychologists such as Rosenhan (1973) have criticized the medical model as being a rationalization for society's use of psychiatry to control deviant behavior. One of the most powerful methods of controlling deviant behavior, they argue, is the process of labeling by psychiatric diagnosis. Merely labeling a person as mentally ill reinforces his deviant role within the community, legitimizes his isolation from the rest of society, and contributes to the stripping from him of his dignity, civil rights, and personal autonomy. Viewed in this context, psychoactive drugs are a further extention of medical labeling. They reinforce the symbolic power of the psychiatrists by giving them chemical control, which leads to the further dehumanization of the individual so-called "patient."

Common to these two schools of criticism is an attack on the basic concept that mental illnesses, including schizophrenia, are appropriately treated within the medical model and that psychiatry and its treatments, be they psychological, such as psychoanalysis, or biological, such as psychoactive drugs, are legitimate medical activities. At its most extreme is Szasz's polemic that mental illness is a myth and that all drugs are chemical straitjackets. In its more mild form, numerous legislative committees and government commissions are investigating the adequacy of checks and balances on the powers of psychiatrists.

It is true that, having separated the mad from the bad, nineteenth-century humanitarians went on to create special institutions called mental hospitals and gave special powers of incarceration to physicians. The authority to label someone as ill is one of the most important parts of the healer role, and there is ample evidence that physicians sometimes overextend and abuse this power. However, it is uncertain whether or not it is possible in a modern society to completely eliminate involuntary hospitalization. Some recent efforts at deinstitutionalization in California and New York seem to have been failures and to have caused more misery for the patients dumped into the community than may have been prevented by eliminating hospitalization. The fact that professions and institutions may abuse at times the power given to them should not necessarily lead us to conclude that the best solution is the anarchic one—to completely eliminate the institution. Our society has, with other professions and other institutions, developed checks and balances to maintain the social functions performed by these institutions while at the same time restricting the potential abuse of power and misuse of authority.

Schizophrenia as a Disease

The basic premise of the disease concept is that a group of behaviors such as those now called schizophrenia are psychopathological. From research evidence and clinical experience it is
concluded that certain of the experiences and behaviors of individuals labeled schizophrenia are abnormal. They are distressing to the individual and to those around him, and are profoundly
maladaptive for the individual in relation to his family and his
social groupings. While there may be similarities and continui-
ties between the schizophrenic's experience and the emotional
life of "normals," by virtue of the intensity of these experiences,
their persistence, and the degree of their interference with the
usual psychological, cognitive, and perceptual norms and with
accepted social behavior, the schizophrenic state is best regarded as an illness, and the disease concept is the most applicable.

This position is opposed to the view of Szasz that mental illness in general, and schizophrenia in particular, is a myth. If it is
a myth, then the individuals who are schizophrenic are doubly
delusional in their suffering. It is also a myth with a genetic
transmission and a pharmacological antidote. This position is
also opposed to that of Laing and many of the family therapists,
who deny that there is such a thing as a patient per se and who
state that the locus of pathology is in the family or in the society
at large. Although there are important familial and social influences upon the eipdemiology of schizophrenia and the life of the
individual schizophrenic, it is a bizzare form of sophistry to deny
the sick role and the opportunity of being treated to the patient
by placing blame on the family or society, as Seigler and Osmond
point out (1974).

I also strongly disagree with the labeling school of sociology
and social psychology, particularly Scheff and Rosenhan, who
say the problems of the schizophrenic are mainly due to the way
in which psychiatrists label him and the society rejects him.
Such processes may indeed go on, but they do not obviate the
inherent difficulties that the schizophrenic experiences in his attempts to find a place for himself in the world.

What has been the influence of the disease approach on understanding schizophrenia? The neo-Kraepelinian answer has been another question: Does the concept of schizophrenia have any meaning, and if it does, what are the data that give it meaning? In other words, the concern has been with what one might call the epistemology of diagnosis; namely, what are the rules of the game?

In the disease approach, there are six steps toward validating a concept of an illness such as schizophrenia.

(1) Define the theoretical bases with clarity. It is very important to make explicit the assumptions on which the many conceptual views of schizophrenia are based. But unfortunately much of psychiatric discourse until the middle of this century has never moved beyond these theoretical debates. In order to move psychiatry beyond philosophy and into science, the second step must be taken.

(2) Translate the general concept into specific hypotheses that can be operationally tested. For example, what is the meaning of borderline schizophrenia? What are its components? How does it manifest itself?

(3) Put the hypothesis to empirical testing to determine its reliability. How well do several observers agree that a borderline patient does have ego deficits, is using splitting or denial?

(4) Subject the data to various statistical tests to determine whether we are dealing with one syndrome alone or a mixture of syndromes.

(5) Attempt to validate the statistics by follow-up studies, family and genetic investigation, correlates in childhood development, and so on.

(6) Undertake epidemiological studies to ascertain the patterns of incidence and prevalence.

How well, then, does schizophrenia meet the criteria of a chronic disease in the medical model? It meets it well but not completely. Before one can conclude definitively that schizophrenia is a disease, conclusive evidence will have to be presented as to etiology and clinical course. While such evidence exists for many other disorders in psychiatry, it does not yet exist for schizophrenia—nor for many other clinical conditions with which medicine deals, such as hypertension, arthritis, and leukemia. That is to say, it is an obviously disordered state with multiple determinants in which there is not certainty as to the exact etiology. Moreover, schizophrenia as we now define it is similar to hypertension in that it is likely to comprise various disorders. As the specific etiological principles come into scientific investigation, we will probably reaffirm Bleuler's concept of a group of schizophrenias. Nevertheless, it is likely that within this group of schizophrenias there is a core group that has a strong genetic component. This genetic factor creates a vulnerability that becomes manifest in psychosis when precipitated by environmental stresses.

I have mentioned that schizophrenia is best understood when viewed as a chronic disease. The chronic disease approach is a subvariant of the classical disease approach, which deals with acute states of relatively short duration such as those brought on by trauma and infection. In contrast, the chronic disease approach contains a number of common features such as mixed etiology, no cure, and long course with intermittent recurrences. The goal in the chronic disease approach is prevention of disability and complications. Most conditions with which medicine deals today are chronic conditions. Some, such as tuberculosis or syphilis, have established etiologies. Syphilitic disease of the brain is one classic example of a chronic illness in psychiatry whose etiology has been elucidated by research in the medical model. But other illnesses show symptom complexes whose boundaries are sometimes difficult to demarcate, but which have generally describable clinical presentation and characteristic course. Nevertheless, within each syndrome there is considerable variation among individual patients. Moreover, there is uncertainty as to whether the group represents a single etiological entity or, as is most likely the case, represents complex multiple etiologies.

An excellent example in psychiatry of such a complex grouping is mental retardation. With the success of biological investigation of the aminoacidurias and chromosomal abnormalities, this large, heterogeneous grouping of mental deficiencies has been broken down. Such a process will soon be underway in schizophrenia. In fact, it has already begun, with the delineation of those schizophrenic syndromes that are due to drugs, such as amphetamines, as distinguished from those that are associated with epilepsy or diseases such as lupus, as well as from differential response to pharmacologic agents.

New Approaches to Diagnosis

The researchers and clincians whom I have referred to as neo-Kraepelinians felt themselves an embattled minority and undertook to devise operational criteria for the diagnosis of schizophrenia and to validate it by follow-up studies and reliability studies. The group from Washington University produced a set of criteria for diagnosis that was published first by Feighner and has become known as the Feighner criteria (Feighner et al. 1972). Later, an expanded version was published, edited by Woodruff, called *Psychiatric Diagnosis* (Woodruff et al. 1974). Next a study was conducted between the Maudsley Hospital in London and the New York State Psychiatric Institute at Columbia, termed the US-UK study (Strauss 1973; Strauss et al. 1974). This large investigation attempted to understand why so much more schizophrenia was reported in the United States than in Great Britain, where a high rate of affective disorders was reported. In addition there was a nine nation study sponsored by the World Health Organization called the International Pilot Study of Schizophrenia.

These three studies in part overlapped. They shared a concept of schizophrenia as an illness and as a syndrome, and they attempted to define a set of manifest symptoms and behaviors readily observable in an interview situation that could be rated quantitatively, and subjected to statistical analysis. Such data could define schizophrenia as a syndrome in a way that did not make any assumptions in the diagnosis as to either etiology or clinical outcome. The WHO and US-UK studies had one investigator in common, John Wing, who is at the Maudsley Hospital. He had clearly annunciated a descriptive syndrome approach and had devised a symptom scale called the Present State Examination (PSE), a quantitative rating of the patient's present clinical state (Wing et al. 1967).

I want to emphasize the common conceptual approach to diagnosis that underlies such efforts. They all seek to define schizophrenia as a symptom constellation or syndrome manifested by directly observable symptoms. It may be correlated with family antecedents or with certain kinds of communication patterns; it may have a certain outcome or it may not. The attempt, nevertheless, is to clearly separate clinical symptoms from other criteria. The US-UK study presented very convincing evidence that American psychiatry's definitions of schizophrenia were very broad and included conditions that British and European psychiatrists would diagnose as personality disorders, mania, or affective disorders.

The most impressive of the studies is the WHO study involving nine countries, including the USSR and Japan. The impressive aspect of this study is that it developed a set of criteria that could be agreed upon by all nine countries. The Present State Examination devised by Wing was translated into the nine languages, and since there was very high interjudge reliability, it was possible to compare the similarities and differences in diagnoses across the countries. They have now completed a two-year follow-up, and even a five-year follow-up for some patients, and there are clear differences in outcome. For example, there are major national differences in the rate at which schizophrenia is becoming a chronic illness; thus although the symptom complex is capable of being defined cross-nationally, it does not in itself lead to the poor outcome that was originally predicted by Kraepelin.

Spitzer, Endicott, and a research group here that included James Barrett, Martin Keller, and myself (Spitzer et al. 1975; Klerman 1977) have used a set of operational criteria that are built on the St. Louis criteria and take into account some of the experiences of the US-UK and WHO studies. These have been codified into some twenty-one diagnostic sets for manifest diagnosis, called the Research Diagnostic Criteria. These criteria, Spitzer has declared, will be embodied in the third edition of the *Diagnostic and Statistical Manual*. As part of the research to validate these criteria, a number of different samples have been collected. So far, the evidence is overwhelming that when psychiatrists and psychologists use the same meanings and operational concepts of the syndrome, use common criteria, and are trained together, particularly using television tapes and quantitative rating scales, then the interjudge reliability in diagnosis is very

very high—from seventy to ninety percent agreement for schizophrenia and the affective disorders. It falls off appreciably, however, for some of the symptom neuroses and for the personality disorders.

The current revival of a scientific approach to psychiatry in general and to schizophrenia in particular has lead to a systematic attempt to define schizophrenia on the basis of a symptoms syndrome and to apply operational criteria to the syndrome. This is part of an overall view that sees mental illness, like other illnesses, as having causes and delineations. The conviction is that in the absence of etiological knowledge, the most fruitful way to proceed is to define, on descriptive clinical grounds, the various syndromes. This will allow us to bring together groups that are relatively homogeneous from a clincial point of view and to examine them for response to treatment or to subject them to genetic or biochemical investigation. In principle, there is no reason why this approach cannot be applied to the search for psychogenic causation in early childhood experience, or to family interaction, or to communication defects, or to social deprivation. There is no reason why this approach cannot be used for the study of non biological treatments such as individual or group psychotherapy or milieu therapy. It is an interesting observation in the history of psychiatry that those investigators who have attempted to apply these procedures most vigorously have had a biological bias to the etiology of schizophrenia and an interest in biological treatments. My own view is that their minority status in the 1950s led them to see themselves as having to pursue an uphill struggle against what they felt to be the entrenched Meyerian domination of the academic centers, the National Institutes of Mental Health leadership in the United States, and the MRC in Great Britain. Whether this will change as the balance of forces shifts will be something for us to observe in the next decade.

DISCUSSION

You have stressed the current concern of the neo-Kraepelinians with presenting symptoms. Will this approach make outcome predictions any better?

Well, there is currently a large controversy as to the state of outcome for schizophrenia. The Strauss papers (Strauss et al. 1974), which are based on the American sample, state that the outcome is not uniformly bad. Strauss and Carpenter have prospectively applied Langfeld's criteria for process versus reactive schizophrenia and also Schneider's criteria. That is one of the characteristics of all these studies that makes them so powerful; the judgments were prospective, that is, they were made at the index episode. Strauss and Carpenter, and others with similar methodologies, argue for multiple outcomes. Specifically, there is no high correlation between social adjustment, psychotic symptoms, neurotic symptoms, and schizophrenia. Each seem to have independent outcomes. For example, a patient can be high on neurotic symptoms, like phobias and bodily complaints, but low on delusions. So, they argue, it is not useful to think of outcome as a single dimension.

On the other hand, the Yale group of Astrachan et al. (1974) have just completed a four-year follow-up of 150 schizophrenics and they report a rather dismal outcome: over fifty percent of that sample is unemployed and ninety percent have continuing symptoms of some sort or another. Yet, there is a ten-year follow-up from a Canadian sample that reports a good outcome. So there is marked variation in outcome studies even with relatively good criteria. The most distressing report is unpublished data from the WHO study; namely, that patients in the less developed countries like Sri Lanka have better outcome than those in the highly developed industrialized countries. The explanation that is being offered is that we are socializing our patients into the sick role, that our great emphasis on after-care and on help such as disability payments all may foster the schizophrenia label. Less developed countries do not have extensive medical and disability programs, and there the patients have better outcomes. This is confirmed by a set of studies by Nancy Waxler (1976, 1977) an anthropologist working with Elliott Mischler who has studied outcomes of schizophrenics in underdeveloped countries and has compared them to patients studied at the Maudsley. Much of this raises the possibility that outcome is not fixed in any inherent process (which was Kraepelin's idea) but may be as much determined by the nature of the social treatment system in which we and the patients are embedded. Such a conclusion is actually quite contrary to the assumption of the generation of Kraepelin and Bleuler that schizophrenia was a fixed entity with an unfolding of some biological destiny independent of environment.

There is much attempt these days to distinguish acute schizophrenia from affective disorders. Do you think this can be done reliably on the basis of the first psychotic episode?

The way you put the question is similar to the kind of thinking that sent our forefathers round and round. If a patient got better he could not be schizophrenic because true schizophrenia meant deterioration or failure to respond to treatment. The syndrome approach, on the other hand, is to define the patient on the basis of the symptom complex and behaviors that they present and to acknowledge that a certain percentage of that group will have the chronic form of the illness. In other words, some patients with Bleuler's syndrome will have Kraepelin's disease. Bleuler *did* define a syndrome. That syndrome can be produced by amphetamines, by cocaine, by hyperparathyroidism, by B_{12} deficiency. It may even be produced by the same genes that produce mania. A certain fraction of that group of people who exhibit Bleuler's syndrome will go on to have the kind of chronic deterioration that Kraepelin described. Now what percentage of people with Bleuler's syndrome have Kraepelin's disease? That is still a matter of much debate. Henry Stack Sullivan distinguished between those who had the syndrome "schizophrenia" and those who had dementia praecox, namely the chronic disabling illness. The neo-Kraepelinian point of view makes the sharp distinction between the syndrome as a mode of presentation and the outcome. Some patients who present the syndrome later respond to lithium or show a complete remission; to my mind predicting who those will be is one of the very large questions that we have to answer.

Perhaps there are other psychoses besides schizophrenia or affective illness?

Certainly. Some people would argue that many acute psychoses are not schizophrenia or affective states. There is a European school who argue that there is a third psychosis, "psychloid" psychosis or "schizophrenaform" psychosis.

Can a neo-Kraepelinian approach take into account family or developmental history?

Not for diagnosis. For diagnosis, the emphasis is upon the presenting symptoms. In order to make the diagnosis, for example, of bipolar affective disease one does not have to know the family history. The criteria for bipolar disease are the current episode of depression with a past history of a mania, independent of family history or future outcome or response to treatment. That constellation *predicts* a high probability of response to lithium and a high probability of a family history.

Don't you think that the strong biases that the neo-Kraepelinian movement is advocating are going to stir up considerable controversy, say with more psychodynamically oriented psychiatry?

I guarantee it will. It is almost inevitable, I think, as the generation of neo-Kraepelinians peaks in academic prominence. The next generation will then rise in rebellion, saying that the neo-Kraepelinians are cold and indifferent to humanistic values, they underemphasize psychotherapy, they are overly statistical. Then there will be a neo-Meyerian revival.

Do you think the neo-Kraepelinians could ever consider the possibly that Bleuler's syndrome might be caused by abnormal developmental processes?

It is an interesting thing that very few of the neo-Kraepelinians are willing to give other than lip service to developmental causation. They are just vitrioloc about it. Maybe there is something in the personality of people who count partridges in pear trees that they do not think that way.

Strauss and Carpenter do write about chronicity, personality, and symptoms as three dimensions that may predict outcome in schizophrenia. Would this at least give us some hope that the symptom approach is not the only one on which a scientific psychiatry may be focused?

I would say that very few of the investigations I have mentioned are personally interested in, or willing to entertain, on principle, a developmental or psychogenic causation to the major psychoses.

Can you comment on "borderline syndrome" from a neo-Kraepelinian orientation?

Well, the evidence is inconsistent. Dr. Kety found that the diagnosis of borderline shows some genetic loading. However, John Gunderson (1977) has conducted a study using discriminant function, in which he does not find any similarity between schizophrenia and borderline. Grinker (1968) has published a follow-up of his borderline series, and only a small percentage of his borderline patients in a five-year follow-up went on to show anything like a schizophrenic outcome. So if you use symptom profile, which is what Gunderson has done, or prospective outcome, which is what Grinker has done, there is no similarity. If you use genetic loading, as in Kety's study, an association is found. There are so many difficulties in comparing these studies—methodology, criteria, and so on, not to mention the entire concept of "boderline." That's worth a whole book in itself.

Can I express a little bit of skepticism? It is unusual, it seems to me to be successful in medicine with an approach that is purely statistical. A syndrome in medicine is usually meant to mean a set of symptoms that powerfully predict the presence of the illness. For example, the combination of bronze skin and diabetes and something that looks like sclerosis, those three signs, when we see them together, very powerfully predict that the patient has hemochromatosis. But to start statistically looking through such a set of phenomena to find a syndrome would be much different. If one looked through all the patients at the Massachusetts General Hospital who had a high blood sugar, one would find very, very few, I think, with the other signs of hemochromatosis. The likelihood of discovering the syndrome with this methodology would be extremely small because the actual conjunction of these three signs is very rare. In other words, using a statistical analysis of all the patients with certain clinical signs, but without a biological cause, and then hoping to find a homogeneous biological group, is a risky business.

Well, that's a very legitimate criticism. Winokur would say that the statistical approach has paid off with respect to bipolar affective disorder. Specifically, Leonard suggested that separating out people with a history of mania from those without mania could define groups of people who turn out to have very different genetic patterns and patterns of response to lithium. Now that has paid off in the affective disorders and perhaps will pay off in schizophrenia. Of course it would be nice if we could unite symptoms and outcome with autopsy findings—as in hemochromatosis—but we do not have that advantage.

Right, so the question is, without the objective validating criteria can the purely statistical approach ever succeed? The hope is that at least these studies can increase the homogeneity of the group so as to facilitate sampling and communication. In effect, Bleuler's syndrome could be partialed out. We know already that syndromes can be due to cocaine, to amphetamines, to vitamin deficiencies. The logic of the partialing out syndromes has been successful, for example, in mental retardation. Currently psychiatry takes the position that if amphetamine toxicity or cocaine poisoning were the etiology, it was *not* schizophrenia. We could just as well call the picture schizophrenia due to cocaine or amphetamines.

REFERENCES

Astrachan, B., A. Meyers, and C. Schwartz. 1974. A follow-up study of schizophrenic patients. *Archives of General Psychiatry* 31:155–160.

Bleuler, E. 1959. Dementia praecox or the group of schizophrenias (1911). Trans. J. Zinkin. New York: International Universities Press.

Fabraga, H., Jr., J. D. Swartz, and C. A. Wallace. 1968. Ethnic differences in psychopathology. *Archives of General Psychiatry* 19:218–226.

Feighner, J. P., E. Robins, S. B. Guze, et al. 1972. Diagnostic criteria for use in psychiatric research. *Archives of General Psychiatry* 26:57–63.

Foucault, M. 1965. *Madness of civilization: a history of insanity in the age of reason.* Trans. R. Howard. New York: Pantheon Books.

Fox, R. C. 1968. Illness. In *International encyclopaedia of social illness,* ed. D. Sills. New York: Free Press.

Grinker, R. R., B. Werble, and R. Drye. 1968. *The borderline syndrome.* New York: Basic Books.

Gunderson, J., and J. Kolb. 1977. Discriminating features of borderline patients. Presented at the American Psychiatric Association meeting, Toronto, Canada, May.

Guze, S. B. 1970. The need for toughmindedness in psychiatric thinking. *Southern Medical Journal* 63:662–671.

Klerman, G. L. 1976. The psychobiology of affective states: the legacy of Adolf Meyer. Presented at the Adolf Meyer Symposium on Psychobiology, Centennial of the Johns Hopkins University, Baltimore, Maryland, March.

_____. 1977a. Mental illness, the medical model and psychiatry. *Journal of Philosophy and Health* (to be published).

_____. 1977b. The neo-Kraepelinian revival in American psychiatry: its history, promise and prospect. Presented at scientific symposium honoring Dr. Eli Robins by the Department of Psychiatry, Washington University School of Medicine, St. Louis, Missouri, May 27–28.

Klerman, G. L., J. Endicott, R. Spitzer, and R. Hirschfield. 1977. Neurotic depressions: a systematic analysis of multiple criteria and multiple meanings. Presented at American Psychiatric Association meeting, Toronto, Canada, May.

Klein, D., and J. Davis. 1969. *Diagnosis and drug treatment of psychiatric disorders.* Maryland: Williams and Wilkins.

Kraepelin, E. 1913. *Psychiatrie.* Barth: Verlag von Johann Ambrosius.

_____. 1919. *Textbook of psychiatry.* Ed. G. M. Robertson. Edinburgh: Livingstone.

Kramer, M. 1969. Cross-national study of diagnosis of the mental disorders: origin of the problem. *American Journal of Psychiatry* (supplement) 125:115—11.

Laing, R. D. 1967. *The politics of experience.* New York: Pantheon Books.

Meyer-Gross, W., E. Slater, and M. Roth. 1969. *Clinical psychiatry*, 3rd ed. London: Bailliere, Tindall, and Cassell.

Parsons, T. 1951. *The Social system.* Illinois: Free Press of Glencoe.

Robins, E. 1977. New Concepts in the diagnosis of psychiatric disorders. *Annual Review of Medicine* 28:67–73.

Rosenhan, D. L. 1973. On being sane in insane places. *Science* 179:250–258.

Scheff, T. 1964. Societal reaction to deviance: ascriptive elements in the psychiatric screening of mental patients in a midwestern state. *Social Problems* 11:401–413.

Seigler, M., and H. Osmond. 1974. *Models of madness, models of medicine.* New York: Macmillan.

Spitzer, R. L., J. Endicott, and E. Robins. 1975. *Research diagnostic criteria.* New York: New York State Department of Mental Hygiene, Biometrics Branch.

Spitzer, R. L., and P. T. Wilson. 1968. A guide to the APA's new diagnostic nomenclature. *American Journal of Psychiatry* 124:1619–1629.

Strauss, J. S. 1973. Diagnostic models and the nature of psychiatric disorder. *Archives of General Psychiatry* 29:445.

Strauss, J. S., and W. T. Carpenter, J. J. Bartko. 1974. The diagnosis and understanding of schizophrenia. *Schizophrenia Bulletin* 11:61–80.

Szasz, T. S. 1961. *The myth of mental illness: foundations of a theory of personal conduct.* New York: Hoeber-Harper.

Waxler, N. E. 1976. Culture and mental illness, a social labeling perspective. *Journal of Nervous and Mental Disease* 159:379–395.

———. 1977. Is mental illness cured in traditional societies? A theoretical analysis. *Culture, Medicine, and Psychiatry.* 1:233–253.

Wing, J. K., J. L. T. Birley, J. E. Cooper, et al. 1967. Reliability of a procedure for measuring and classifying present psychiatric state. *British Journal of Psychiatry* 113:499–515.

Winokur, G., P. Clayton, and T. Reich. 1969. *Manic-depressive illness.* St. Louis: C. V. Mosby.

Woodruff, R. A., D. W. Goodwin, and S. B. Guze. 1974. *Psychiatric diagnosis.* New York: Oxford University Press.

6

Biochemical Investigation

IAN CREESE AND SOLOMON H. SNYDER

Although it is widely assumed that a biochemical abnormality exists in schizophrenia, no such specific abnormality has yet been established with certainty. The obvious location for such a deficit is within the brain, but since the central nervous system in humans is, of course, not readily accessible to biochemical investigations, the first systematic work on the biochemistry of schizophrenia involved attempts to isolate abnormal substances in the blood or urine of patients. Early studies appeared to indicate the presence of a protein in the serum of schizophrenics that could apparently cause hallucinations if administered to normal volunteers. However, this early experiment was never replicated, and in general any alterations in the blood of schizophrenics appear to be more related to their long periods of institutionalization rather than to their psychotic disturbances (Kety 1959). Chromatographic analysis of the urine of schizophrenics also isolated a chemical that appeared specific to them. Termed the pink spot because of its chromatographic staining properties, it was tentatively identified as 3,4-dimethoxyphenylethylamine, a substance related both to the neurotransmitter dopamine and to the hallucinogenic drug mescaline (Friedhoff and Van Winkle 1963). This identification had obvious appeal. However, further work demonstrated that the pink spot was, in fact, composed of many compounds, including metabolites of antischizophrenic drugs the patients were treated with (Siegel and Tefft 1971; Perry, Hansen, and MacDougall 1967).

Another promising approach in recent years has been the study of certain pharmacologic agents that produce very specific alterations in schizophrenic behavior. Two groups of drugs with diametrically opposed actions on schizophrenic patients are the amphetamines and the neuroleptics. Whereas amphetamines will exacerbate the schizophrenic psychosis, neuroleptics (such as Thorazine and Haldol) specifically relieve psychosis. Much research has been conducted on these drugs in order to discover their biochemical mechanisms of action. Of what use is it to know whether the clinical effects of such drugs derive from one or another biochemical influence? The obvious answer is that if we know the biochemical action of such drugs, we may gain insight into the aberrations that account for the schizophrenic symptoms they relieve. Such an assertion involves certain assumptions, the most crucial being that the drugs are specific in their interaction with schizophrenia. One can readily conceive of an antischizophrenic drug that would make life more livable for schizophrenics and for the staff of mental hospitals without doing anything fundamental to the schizophrenic process. For many years sedatives, straitjackets, and wet sheets have eased the predicaments of schizophrenics and their keepers, but few people would argue that these treatments did anything fundamental to schizophrenic mechanisms. However, amphetamines and neuroleptics do indeed interact specifically and antagonistically with the schizophrenic syndrome.

It has been known for a long time that amphetamines in small doses can exacerbate schizophrenic symptoms. In fact, this observation has even been used as a diagnostic tool. If a diagnosis was questionable, the physician would give the patient a little amphetamine, and if it made him worse rapidly, that would favor a diagnosis of schizophrenia. More recently, John Davis has shown that small intravenous doses of amphetamines or related agents dramatically exacerbate the symptoms of schizophrenia (Janowsky et al. 1973). This exacerbation does not appear to be a manifestation of new symptoms but a worsening of the patient's own psychosis. This effect of amphetamines is not found in manic-depressive patients, neurotics, or persons with other mental illnesses nor in normal healthy controls. However, if people without any schizophrenic disposition take very large doses of amphetamine or become chronic amphetamine abusers, acute paranoid psychoses often occur that are clinically indistinguishable from paranoid schizophrenic episodes (Connell 1958).

Biochemical studies indicate that amphetamines exert their clinical actions by increasing the amount of the neurotransmitters norepinephrine and dopamine in the synaptic cleft. This appears to result from amphetamine's ability to both stimulate the release of the neurotransmitters and also block their specific reuptake mechanisms. Experiments using amphetamine analogues with differential effects on the dopamine and norepinephrine systems suggest that the exacerbation of psychosis is more likely to be mediated through dopamine rather than norepinephrine systems (Snyder et al. 1974). One would thus expect that L-dopa, which is used routinely in parkinsonian patients to raise dopamine levels, would also worsen schizophrenic symptoms. And in fact, several clinical studies have shown that it does (Angrist et al. 1973).

The use of amphetamine psychosis in humans as a model for schizophrenia has been questioned on the ground that individuals with amphetamine psychosis do not display all the abnormalities of thought and action typical of schizophrenia. However, one can consider the pathology of amphetamine psychosis as similar to that of schizophrenia without regarding it as identical. For example, the fact that amphetamine is acting on a nonschizophrenic who knows that the episode is likely to be transient should, in itself, make for major differences. Schizophrenics, by contrast, have been experiencing more or less abnormal mental status for months or years with little or no hope of major relief. Although as of yet no convincing animal model of schizophrenia has been discovered, the administration of amphetamines to rats does produce behaviors that are similar to those seen in human amphetamine addicts. The stereotyped compulsive behaviors seen in such addicts consist of taking things apart, putting them back together, going to the refrigerator, opening it, taking food out, putting it back in, closing it, going back again, taking something apart, putting it back together, and so on. Such behavior has its parallel in rats that have been given amphetamines: they constantly sniff and rear over the same spot in their cage or continuously chew and lick at a certain bar in the cage wall (Randrup and Munkvad 1970). The fact that such amphetamine-induced stereotyped behavior is antagonized by the neuroleptic drugs in both humans and rats and the fact that the relative potencies of the neuroleptics parallel their potencies as antipsychotic agents further reinforce the parallel between amphetamine psychosis and schizophrenia (Janssen and Van Bever 1975).

Chlorpromazine, the first of the phenothiazine neuroleptic drugs, was introduced into clinical practice by Delay and Deniker in 1952. Although chlorpromazine was a powerful sedating agent that quieted hyperactive patients, it paradoxically activated withdrawn patients, suggesting that it was acting selectively on the fundamental schizophrenic abnormality. By contrast, classical sedatives such as phenobarbital sedate all patients alike. The great clinical success of chlorpromazine sparked a large number of inquiries into the biochemical effects of the drug, and the phenothiazine molecule was subjected to numerous remodelings by medicinal chemists (fig. 6.1). The resulting compounds vary in their clinical efficacy. In brief, considering

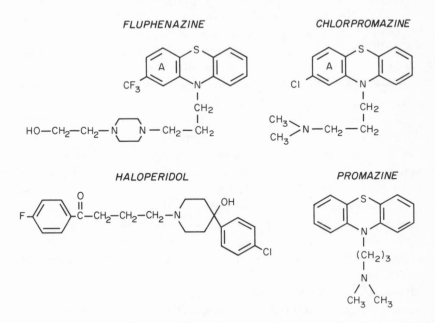

Fig. 6.1. Molecular structures of the phenothiazines fluphenazine, chlorpromazine, and promazine and the butyrophenone haloperidol.

only a few of the numerous derivatives, fluphenazine (Prolixin), with an [F] substituted A ring, is about ten times more potent than chlorpromazine (Thorazine), with a [Cl] substituted A ring, which is many times more potent than promazine (Sparine), with no substitution, which has hardly any antischizophrenic activity. Promethazine (Phenergan) is a similar drug that lacks antischizophrenic activity but, like other efficacious phenothiazines, possesses a full complement of antihistamine side effects (Klein and Davis 1969).

These results are of importance to pharmacologists and biochemists. Such a series of drugs with differing potencies as antipsychotics can be tested in any biochemical system that might be thought to be involved in their therapeutic action. If and when the therapeutically relevant system is investigated, the same relative potencies of the various drugs must be maintained. Drugs such as promazine and promethazine are thus the exceptions which prove the rule in that they possess all the nonspecific side effects of the phenothiazines but none of the critical aspects responsible for the antipsychotic property of the rest of their family. Thus, any biochemical or behavioral test in which promazine is found to be equal to or more potent than chlorpromazine cannot be related directly to the mechanism of action of antipsychotic neuroleptic drugs nor by implication to the schizophrenic process. The phenothiazines are biochemically highly reactive drugs and have been shown to influence numerous enzyme and membrane properties. However, most of these studies failed to demonstrate the correct potency ordering of the various members of the phenothiazine family; moreover, many of the effects occurred only at very high drug concentrations unlikely to be achieved in the clinical situation.

Phenothiazines antagonize amphetamine-induced stereotyped behavior in rats (Randrup and Munkvad 1970). Moreover, another class of neuroleptic agents, the butyrophenones, of which haloperidol (Haldol) is a well known example (fig. 6.1), are antipsychotic and also block amphetamine-induced stereotyped behavior in rats. Although there is little similarity in the structure of phenothiazines and butyrophenones, their similar behavioral effects prompted consideration that they might both act by the same mechanism, namely, blocking the effects of dopamine in the brain (Janssen and Van Bever 1975).

How did this hypothesis arise? Neuroleptics produce a cataleptic or akinetic syndrome in rats, similar to the syndrome of Parkinson's disease, that is related to a depletion of dopamine. Thus, it was hypothesized that the neuroleptics might act by depleting brain levels of dopamine. However, when this was investigated experimentally, Carlsson found that not only was there no change in dopamine levels but that the levels of dopamine metabolites were significantly increased (Carlsson and Lindqvist 1963). Carlsson attempted to reconcile this finding of normal levels of dopamine and elevated values of metabolites with a hypothetical "functional deficiency of dopamine." He reasoned that the increase in metabolite production, along with normal levels of dopamine, suggested that the drug treatments provoked an enhanced synthesis and release of dopamine. Since neurotransmitter synthesis usually parallels the activity of neurons, it might be inferred that dopamine neurons fire more rapidly after neuroleptic treatment. But accelerated firing of neurons with transmitter release should result in hyperactivity of the total system rather than a deficiency. Not so, Carlsson conjectured, since one way drugs could speed the firing of neurons while decreasing synaptic effects would be by blocking postsynaptic receptors. Somehow a message from the postsynaptic neuron would convey information, via interneurons, back to the dopamine neuron to the effect that "we are not receiving enough dopamine, turn on the dopamine machine." The dopamine neurons would then increase their firing rate in order to compensate for the functional block of dopamine neurotransmission. With more dopamine being released, catabolism would lead to the elevated metabolite levels. However, with the drug sitting on the dopamine receptors, the released dopamine would not be able to exert its normal effects.

Many subsequent experiments, both pharmacologic and neurophysiologic, have demonstrated conclusively that the neuroleptics do indeed accelerate the firing of dopamine neurons (Bunney et al. 1973). Demonstrating that they also block dopamine receptor sites, however, has proved much more difficult, and for a long time much of the evidence was indirect. The first direct approach to this was by Paul Greengard at Yale, who found that there was an adenylate cyclase located in the striatum, a dopamine rich region of the brain, which was selectively stimulated by dopamine (Kebabian et al. 1972). This selective sensitivity to dopamine led to the hypothesis that the adenylate cyclate was associated with the dopamine receptor. The fact that phenothiazines blocked this enzyme with some correlation with their clinical efficacy further supported this hypothesis. However, later research led to problems. Figure 6.2 shows the relative potencies of neuroleptics in humans as antipsychotics and their affinities for inhibiting the dopamine-sensitive adenylate cyclase (using the more extensive data of Iversen et al. 1976). There is no statistically significant correlation when all the different groups of neuroleptics are considered, even though there is a correlation among the phenothiazines when considered alone (Snyder et al. 1975). The problem lies with the butyrophenones, such as haloperidol, which are very potent clinically but which are very weak in this *in vitro* system. In fact, because they are so weak at inhibiting the dopamine-sensitive adenylate cyclase, many investigators speculated that the butyrophenones must act by a different mechanism and do not block dopamine receptors. This result brought into question the whole dopamine hypothesis of schizophrenia. We therefore investigated the binding of radioactively labeled haloperidol to brain membranes to see if haloperidol did, in fact, bind to dopamine receptors.

Identification of neurotransmitter receptors is a young science, dating from 1970, when several groups succeeded in labeling the nicotinic acetylcholine receptor in certain electric fish. Their success was due in part to the availability of radioactively labeled snake venom toxins which, once bound to the receptor, remained attached. Progress in labeling receptors in the brain was hampered by the fact that both neurotransmitters and their antagonists are rather loosely bound to receptor sites, making it hard to distinguish specific receptor binding from nonspecific absorption. Only recently has this problem been overcome by using low concentrations of ligands (the neurotransmitter or drugs that bind to the receptor) labeled to high specific activity, followed by rapid and vigorous washing of the tissue to remove nonspecifically bound molecules.

In binding studies of any neurotransmitter receptor one cannot reiterate too often that certain criteria must be satisfied before concluding that the binding site is the biologically relevant re-

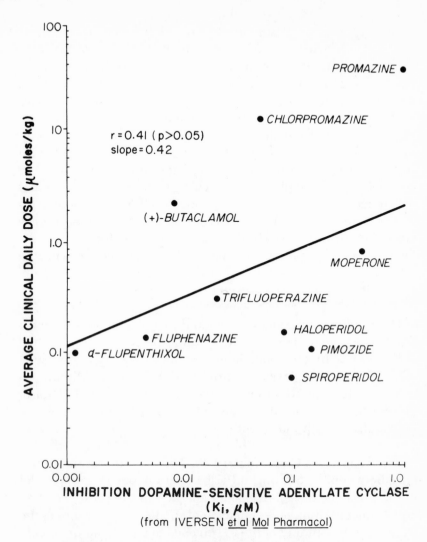

Fig. 6.2. Lack of a significant correlation among antischizophrenic drugs between affinities for inhibition of the dopamine-sensitive adenylate cyclase (from Iversen et al. 1976) and clinical potencies ($r = 0.41$, $p > 0.05$) (from Snyder et al. 1975).

ceptor. These are (1) saturability: radiolabeled ligand binding must saturate with increasing concentrations of radiolabeled ligand, indicating that the binding sites are finite in number; (2) regional localization: binding sites should be found only in areas where the neurotransmitter itself is present (although this does not necessarily imply a perfect correlation between the level of neurotransmitter and the concentration of its receptor sites in various brain areas); and most importantly (3) pharmacological specificity: agonists and antagonists that differ in potencies in *in vivo* behavioral and pharmacological tests should exhibit parallel differences in potency in competing for the radio-labeled ligand's binding sites. This last criterion takes on added importance if optical isomers of a drug have markedly different behavioral and clinical potencies. Their abilities to interact with the relevant neurotransmitter receptor must also exhibit isomeric specificity and thus can be used to define stereospecific receptor binding.

The binding of [^{3}H]haloperidol and that of another antagonist butyrophenone, [^{3}H]spiroperidol, fulfill the conditions outlined above for labeling the dopamine receptor in the brain (Creese et al. 1975). Specific [^{3}H]haloperidol binding is saturable and reversible with a dissociation constant of 1-2 nM, while [^{3}H]spiroperidol has a dissociation constant of 0.2 nM. Butaclamol is a new antischizophrenic agent that exists as optical isomers, with virtually all the dopamine blocking activity residing in the (+) isomer (Voith and Cummings 1976). Thus, the maximum difference between the binding of [^{3}H]haloperidol or [^{3}H]spiroperidol in the presence of (+)butaclamol and that in the presence of an equal concentration of (−)butaclamol should be a measure of the stereospecific binding of the [^{3}H]ligands to the dopamine receptor (fig. 6.3). Although a low concentration of [^{3}H]haloperidol clearly binds to several high affinity sites, probably including alpha-adrenergic receptors as well as dopamine receptors, the portion of binding that is delineated by the stereospecific displacement by the isomers of butaclamol appears to have the pharmacologic characteristics of binding to the dopamine receptor (Burt et al. 1976b).

We have also been able to use the neurotransmitter itself, [^{3}H]dopamine, to label dopamine receptors (Burt et al. 1976b).

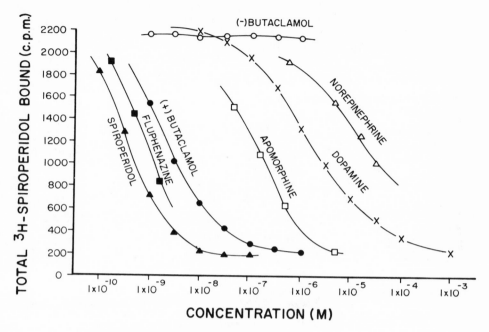

Fig. 6.3. Competition of drugs for binding of [³H]spiro-peridol. Increasing concentrations of nonradioactive drugs were added to tubes containing 0.15 nM [³H] spiroperidol and rat striatal membranes. Bound radioactivity was separated by filtration.

For both [³H]dopamine and [³H]haloperidol binding sites, (+)bu-taclamol is about one hundred and one thousand times more potent, respectively, than the clinically inactive (−)isomer. Other known dopamine agonists and antagonists reduce the [³H]ligands' binding competitively to the same extent as the high affinity component of the displacement by (+)butaclamol. The maximum high affinity components are not additive, indicating that these drugs are competing for the same class of [³H]ligand binding sites. Seeman's group in Toronto has also characterized dopamine receptor binding with these [³H]ligands (Seeman et al. 1975).

The relative potencies of other dopamine agonists and antagonists in competing for [³H]dopamine, [³H]haloperidol, and [³H]spiroperidol binding are similar, which supports the hypothesis that these ligands bind to the same receptor. Apomorphine is the agonist with the highest affinity for all ligands, somewhat greater than that of dopamine itself. Dopamine is more than ten times as potent as norepinephrine; isoproterenol, the most active catecholamine at beta receptors, is essentially inactive. This series closely parallels the ability of these agents to stimulate the dopamine-sensitive adenylate cyclase. Among the neuroleptic dopamine antagonists there is a general correlation with pharmacologic potencies for the phenothiazines at both dopamine and haloperidol sites: fluphenazine is more active than chlorpromazine, which is more active than promazine and promethazine.

One of the major items of evidence that [³H]dopamine and [³H]haloperidol bind to the same dopamine receptors derives from regional studies. The [³H]ligands display very similar regional variations in binding. High binding for both ligands occurs in the caudate nucleus of the calf brain, with lesser amounts in the globus pallidus, putamen, olfactory tubercle, and nucleus accumbens. Receptor binding has not been detected in areas such as the hippocampus and cerebellum, where there is no known dopamine innervation (Burt et al. 1976b). We have recently detected binding in the pituitary, where the receptor sites may be involved in the control of prolactin release (Creese, Schneider, and Snyder 1977). The pituitary dopamine receptors appear to have a very similar drug specificity to the dopamine receptors in the brain.

If one looks more closely at drug affinity for [³H]dopamine binding sites, one finds some relation to clinical potency among the phenothiazines (table 6.1). Fluphenazine is more potent than chlorpromazine, and promazine is definitely weaker. Although they are in the right order, we should note that the clinical differences among these drugs are considerably greater than their differences in competing for [³H]dopamine binding. However, when we consider the butyrophenones such as haloperidol, we find that they are weaker than would be expected from clinical data, as we found with antagonizing the dopamine-sensitive adenylate cyclase. What is the explanation for this result? If both [³H]dopamine and [³H]haloperidol binding and the dopamine-sensitive adenylate cyclase are all markers of the same dopamine receptor, we should expect to find the same affinity for any drug in all three systems.

Table 6.1. Displacement of specific [³H]dopamine and [³H]haloperidol binding from calf striatal membranes.[a]

	K_i,nM [³H]dopamine binding		K_i,nM [³H]haloperidol binding	
Dopamine	17.5 ±	0.9	670	± 80
Apomorphine	8.6 ±	0.5	51	± 8
Norepinephrine	200 ±	19	5,600	± 530
Isoproterenol	>10,000		>10,000	
(+)-Butaclamol	80 ±	11	0.54 ±	0.08
(−)-Butaclamol	>10,000		700	± 120
α-Flupenthixol	180 ±	30	0.98 ±	0.11
β-Flupenthixol	8,000 ±	900	48	± 15
cis-Thiothixene	540 ±	140	1.5 ±	0.10
trans-Thiothixene	15,000	± 2,100	145	± 41
Fluphenazine	230 ±	30	0.88 ±	0.12
Chlorpromazine	900 ±	200	10.2 ±	1.6
Promazine	7,100	± 1,600	72	± 3
Promethazine	12,000	± 3,600	240	± 30
Spiroperidol	1,400 ±	190	0.25 ±	0.02
Pimozide	5,300	± 1,100	0.81 ±	0.09
Haloperidol	920 ±	90	1.4 ±	0.10

[a] Fresh or frozen calf striatal membranes were assayed by filtration with three or more concentrations of each drug in triplicate. IC_{50} values were determined by log-probit plots and converted to K_i's according to the formula $K_i = IC_{50}/(1+c/K_D)$, where c is the concentration of radioactive drug (5 nM for [³H]dopamine and 2 nM for [³H]haloperidol) and K_D is 20 nM for dopamine binding and 2 nM for haloperidol binding. Each value listed is the mean of at least three determinations.

A possible explanation has grown out of work with other neurotransmitter receptors such as the opiate, serotonin, muscarinic-cholinergic, glycine, and the alpha-noradrenergic receptors. Such work has made it very clear that neurotransmitters themselves (which are agonists) bind in a very different way from antagonists. It appears that neurotransmitter receptors can exist in two discrete states, one favoring the binding of agonists and the other favoring the binding of antagonists (Snyder 1975a). Table 6.1 shows us what happens at the dopamine receptor. Notice that agonists like dopamine and apomorphine are more potent in competing for [³H]dopamine binding than [³H]haloperidol binding (the smaller the number the more potent the drug). Dopamine is three hundred times more potent competing for [³H]dopamine binding than competing for [³H]haloperidol binding. In the case of the antagonists we find the exact opposite: haloperidol is hundreds of times more potent when competing for [³H]haloperidol binding than for [³H]dopamine binding. Spiroperidol is six thousand times more potent competing for [³H]haloperidol binding than for [³H]dopamine binding. Clearly, antagonists have a greater affinity for [³H]haloperidol binding, while agonists have a greater affinity for [³H]dopamine binding (Burt et al. 1976b).

Our studies of the opiate/enkephalin receptor demonstrated that the agonist and antagonist states of the receptor are directly interconvertible and are under the allosteric influence of sodium and manganese ions (Snyder 1975b). Increasing the concentration of sodium in the medium decreases the number of agonist sites while concurrently increasing the number of antagonist sites. Manganese ions work in the opposite direction. In this case, agonist and antagonist states of the receptor are hypothesized to exist in equilibrium. Such a model can explain much of the data. For instance, why is an antagonist an antagonist? It has been traditionally thought that an agonist is a drug that approaches the receptor, is recognized, binds, and then triggers some change in ion permeability. An antagonist approaches the same receptor, is recognized, binds, but triggers no further change. The fact that the antagonist is already occupying the receptor prevents the approach of further agonist molecules, thus blocking their effects. However, in the two-state model, as shown in figure 6.4, the pharmacological effects of antagonists occur not by directly blocking agonist access to receptor sites but indirectly, by binding to the antagonist states of the receptor and decreasing the number of agonist states available by causing them to interconvert to antagonist states to reestablish the equilibrium between the two states. This model also explains how neurotransmitter recognition is translated into an alteration in ion conductance. The appropriate ion, in this case sodium, is postulated to have selective affinity for the antagonist state of the receptor. In its resting condition the receptor is largely in the antagonistic binding state because of the high levels of body so-

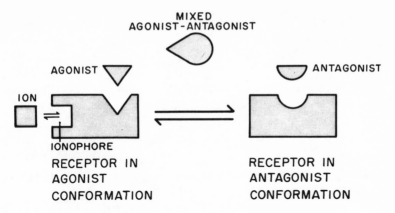

Fig. 6.4. Two-state model of receptor action (from Snyder 1975a).

dium. When the neurotransmitter binds to the receptor, it transforms a portion of the receptor into the agonist state and thus the binding of the crucial ion also changes, eliciting the appropriate change in conductance. Recent electrophysiological evidence bolsters this hypothesis by implicating changes in sodium conductance as a major synaptic mechanism of opiate action. In the case of the glycine receptor, synaptic action is mediated by changes in chloride conductance, and chloride ions have been shown to influence directly interconvertible binding states of the receptor (Snyder 1975a).

Although we have yet to directly demonstrate ionic influences on the serotonin, dopamine, or muscarinic cholinergic receptors, it is apparent that agonist and antagonist binding sites may also exist for these receptors. A prediction of this model is that if one has a mixed agonist–antagonist drug (which is also called a partial agonist), it should have similar affinity for the two states of the receptor. In the dopamine system there is actually such a drug, and it is the well known substance lysergic acid diethylamide (LSD). In behavioral studies LSD displays dopaminergic activity, like apomorphine (Pieri et al. 1974). LSD will also stimulate the dopamine-sensitive adenylate cyclase in the striatum, but it mimics neuroleptics as well, in that it will block the actions of dopamine (Von Hungen et al. 1975). Thus, it is both an agonist and an antagonist. If our model is valid, LSD should demonstrate similar affinity for the two states of the receptor. As is shown in table 6.2, LSD had in essence the same affinity for both [³H]dopamine and [³H]haloperidol binding (Burt et al. 1976a; 1976b). Notice that the effects are very stereospecific; d-LSD is thousands of times more potent than l-LSD. This is interesting because the psychedelic actions of LSD are stereospecific, too. Thus, stereospecificity is not necessarily restricted to one action of the drug.

How the two-state model should be visualized at the molecular level is still uncertain and will probably remain so until someone succeeds in actually determining the structure of a receptor site. It may involve a stereochemical change in the receptor or, alternatively, it may involve two adjacent molecules or adjacent sites on the same receptor molecule, one binding agonists and the other binding antagonists. Additional models are also possible, but with the present state of knowledge there seems little point in speculating about them.

What is the clinical relevance of this data? Now that we can measure the dopamine receptor and its antagonist state, let us

Table 6.2. Inhibition of [³H]dopamine and [³H]haloperidol binding by LSD.[a]

Drug	K_i,nM [³H]dopamine	K_i,nM [³H]haloperidol
Dopamine	20	600
Apomorphine	8	60
d-LSD	29	20
l-LSD	50,000	20,000
Fluphenazine	160	1.3
Haloperidol	800	2

[a] For each drug listed competition for binding of both ligands was measured at three or more concentrations of drug, and the concentration that inhibited binding by 50%, the IC_{50}, was derived by log-probit analysis. Binding of [³H]dopamine was independently determined (by Scatchard plots) to have a K_D of about 20 nM, while that of [³H]haloperidol was about 2 nM. These values were used to convert IC_{50} values to apparent K_i's (inhibition constants) according to the equation $K_i = IC_{50}/ (1+C/K_D)$, where C is the concentration of radioactive ligand (5 nM for [³H]dopamine and 2 nM for [³H]haloperidol). Each value listed is the mean of at least three determinations.

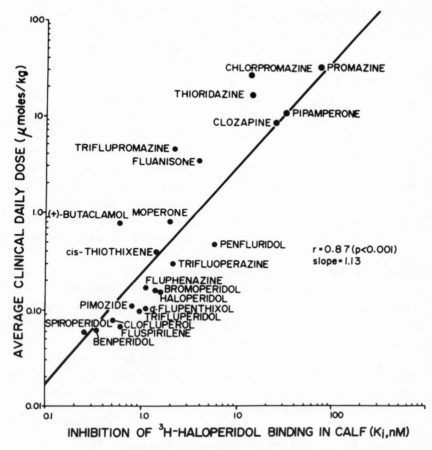

Fig. 6.5. Correlation among antischizophrenic drugs between affinities for [³H]haloperidol binding and clinical potencies. Clinical data were derived from published results. Mean of each daily dose range listed for each drug was meaned and converted to moles/kg assuming a human body weight of 70 kg. The correlation coefficient $r = 0.87$ is significant at the $p < 0.001$ level. (From Creese et al. 1976b.)

see how clinical potencies of neuroleptic drugs correlate with their affinities for the dopamine receptor. Figure 6.5 shows that clinical potency as measured by the daily average dose for antipsychotic activity correlates very well ($r = 0.87$, $p < 0.001$) with affinity for the dopamine receptor (Creese et al. 1976a; 1976b).

This is all the more incredible because clinical doses of any one neuroleptic vary so widely depending on many factors such as the psychiatrist, the institution, and so on. One might argue that the reason all the points fall on a straight line is because we have adjusted the doses to make them fit. So let us try something a little more rigorous, such as the ability of neuroleptics to block apomorphine-induced stereotyped behavior in rats, where molar potency can be quantified exactly. Figure 6.6 shows that the same very high correlation is found. What about other behaviors that are even more relevant to schizophrenia? For example, amphetamine psychosis certainly mimics schizophrenic behavior in some respects. Does the ability of a neuroleptic drug to antagonize amphetamine-induced stereotyped behavior in rats correlate with its affinity for the dopamine receptor? Figure 6.7 shows that it correlates very well. This kind of direct data gives us confidence that we are in fact dealing with the dopamine receptor and, even more relevantly, that the therapeutic action of neuroleptic drugs in schizophrenia is associated with a blockade of dopamine receptors. Indeed, this correlation between biochemical effects in a test tube and therapeutic action is a better correlation than one would get from most other drugs in general use today. In terms of determining the mechanism of drug action, in this case psychiatry and psychopharmacology stand up pretty well.

There is more that we can learn from these binding studies on rats. We know a great deal about dopamine in terms of its pathways and behavioral effects that may be relevant to a number of clinical phenomena. One interesting aspect of the dopamine neuronal system is that it is uncrossed, so that dopamine cell bodies in the left substantia nigra innervate the left striatum only. If 6-hydroxydopamine is injected into the surrounding area of the substantia nigra, it selectively accumulates in the dopamine cell bodies and since 6-hydroxydopamine is neurotoxic, the dopamine cells are selectively destroyed. Injection on one side of the brain thus causes a unilateral denervation of the ipsilateral striatum. Since one of the functions of the striatum is to regulate motor activity, the unilateral nigrostriatal lesion leads to an asymmetry in the striatal input. Thus, if the rat is given amphetamine, which releases dopamine from the intact terminals on the unlesioned side, the animal shows a marked motor asymmetry

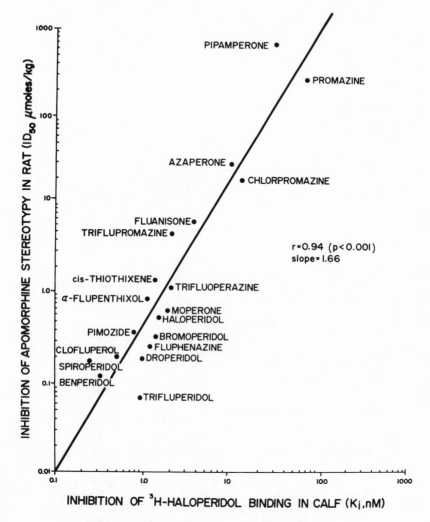

Fig. 6.6. Correlation among neuroleptic drugs between affinities for [³H]haloperidol bindings sites and antagonism of apomorphine stereotypy in the rat. Animal data were derived from published results and converted to moles/kg. The correlation coefficient $r = 0.94$ is significant at the $p < 0.001$ level.

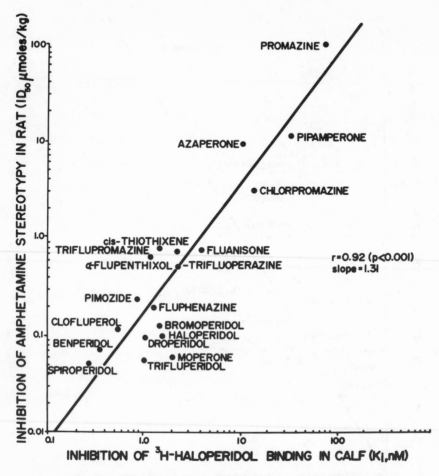

Fig. 6.7. Correlation among neuroleptic drugs between
affinities for [³H]haloperidol binding sites and antagonism of amphetamine stereotypy in the rat. Animal data
were derived from published results and converted to
moles/kg. The correlation coefficient $r = 0.92$ is significant at the $p < 0.001$ level.

and rotates towards the side of the lesion because there is no dopamine being released from the side that is lesioned (Creese,
Burt, and Snyder 1977). One might expect that if one gave apomorphine, which stimulates dopamine receptors directly, no
asymmetry would result, since one has not lesioned the recep-

tors themselves on either side. However, such rats given apomorphine rotate in the opposite direction to that after amphetamine administration (Ungerstedt 1971). This indicates that the receptors on the lesioned side of the brain have become hypersensitive to the effects of apomorphine. Such an effect has been termed "behavioral supersensitivity." We have been interested in investigating whether this phenomenon is indeed the result of a true increase in receptor sensitivity following denervation. This is of clinical importance: in Parkinson's disease the nigrostriatal pathway also degenerates (caused by some unknown mechanism), and the efficacy of L-dopa therapy seems, in part, to arise through an enhanced sensitivity to this dopamine agonist in such patients.

When we compared the binding of [³H]haloperidol in the lesioned striatum to that in the unlesioned striatum in the same rat, we found that indeed there was a marked increase in the number of receptors on the lesioned side (Creese, Burt, and Snyder 1977). However, there was no apparent change in the binding affinity for [³H]haloperidol. If this increase in receptor number is responsible for the enhanced behavioral effects of apomorphine, then one would expect that the larger the increase in receptor numbers the greater the number of rotations that would be caused by apomorphine in the same animal. Figure 6.8 shows that animals with the greatest increase in receptor numbers show the greatest number of rotations to apomorphine.

Drug-induced receptor supersensitivity may be responsible for a troubling side effect that arises in the treatment of schizophrenics, namely tardive dyskinesia. Tardive dyskinesia, which occurs after the chronic treatment of schizophrenics with neuroleptics for a period of months, is characterized by constant movements of the mouth and lips and protrusion of the tongue, sometimes leading to difficulties in eating and breathing (Kobayashi 1977). Choreiform movements of the arms may also occur. Paradoxically, when neuroleptic administration is stopped, the symptoms get worse, but diminish when the dose of the neuroleptic is increased. However, after a short time at the new higher dose level, the symptoms reappear. Interestingly, these symptoms of tardive dyskinesia resemble the effects of an overdose of L-dopa in parkinsonian patients. It has thus been hypothesized that tar-

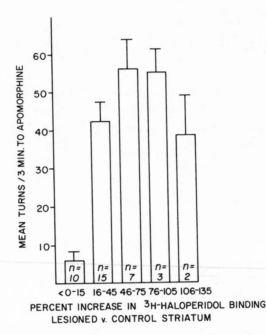

Fig. 6.8. Correlation between increased [³H]haloperidol binding in the lesioned striatum and behavioral super-sensitivity to apomorphine following unilateral nigro-striatal 6-hydroxydopamine lesion. Rotational behavior to apomorphine (0.25 mg/kg s.c.) was measured between two and seven months after unilateral injection of 6-hy-droxydopamine into the substantia nigra. Striatal [³H]ha-loperidol binding was assayed in the lesioned and con-trol striatum of each rat separately between one and ten weeks later and is expressed as the mean ratio of spe-cific c.p.m. [³H]haloperidol bound in the lesioned/con-trol striatum at 4 concentrations of [³H]haloperidol (0.4–4.0 nM). Each data point represents an individual rat.

dive dyskinesia results from a functional excess of dopamine ac-tivity (Klawans 1973). It is as if blocking the dopamine receptors over a long period of time causes them to fight back, to hypertro-phy, so that they become behaviorally supersensitive to dopa-mine. But the behavioral supersensitivity could be due to com-pensatory changes occuring in other neuronal pathways or to a biochemical mechanism such as an increase in enzyme activity.

To examine whether tardive dyskinesia is really related to a change in the number of dopamine receptor sites, we looked at a simple animal model that was developed by Tarsy and Baldessarini (1974). The behavioral sensitivity of dopamine receptors was tested by giving rats apomorphine and quantifying the doses that lead to stereotyped behavior. A neuroleptic was then given for a number of weeks, after which it was stopped and the rats were tested again with apomorphine. A lower dose of apomorphine was then found to induce the stereotyped behavior indicating behavioral supersensitivity had developed. After treating rats on similar dose schedules of fluphenazine or haloperidol for three weeks, we found an increase in [^{3}H]haloperidol binding of twenty to twenty-five percent five days after terminating the chronic treatment (Burt et al. 1977). This increase in the amount of dopamine receptor binding could be due to an increase in the number of binding sites or to a change in the affinity of the receptors for [^{3}H]haloperidol. Scatchard analysis of the binding data indicated that in fact there was an increase in the number of dopamine receptors. This increase is not as great, however, as the behavioral supersensitivity, which indicates that there may be some amplifying mechanism involved. Nonetheless, it may be possible with this approach to evaluate biochemically different drugs to determine which of them might have a greater propensity for producing tardive dyskinesia.

Studying the influences of neuroleptics on other neurotransmitter receptors can give us important information about other aspects of their clinical pharmacology. For instance, neuroleptics vary in their propensity to elicit extrapyramidal parkinsonian-like side effects such as rigidity and akinesia. It has been hypothesized that dopamine receptor blockade in the corpus striatum is responsible for these extrapyramidal side effects, while dopamine receptor blockade in the limbic forebrain region is responsible for the antischizophrenic efficacy of neuroleptic agents (Snyder et al. 1974). However, regional studies of [^{3}H]haloperidol binding have not indicated any fundamental differences in dopamine receptor binding between the corpus striatum, limbic, or cortical areas, even for neuroleptics such as thioridazine and clozapine which have much lower incidence of extrapyramidal side effects (Burt et al. 1976b).

Recent studies of the muscarinic-cholinergic receptor in the brain have provided a resolution of this dilemma. It is well known that concurrent administration of anticholinergic drugs is especially effective in antagonizing the extrapyramidal side effects of neuroleptics without apparently reducing their antipsychotic potencies. The therapeutic efficacy of anticholinergics apparently reflects a balance between dopamine and acetycholine in the corpus striatum. Thus, antagonizing acetycholine effects is equivalent to enhancing those of dopamine and vice versa (Snyder et al. 1974). We reasoned that if neuroleptics vary in their anticholinergic propensities, they might vary in their propensity to induce extrapyramidal side effects. In studies of the binding of [^{3}H]QNB, a potent antagonist at muscarinic-cholinergic receptors, to striatal membrane preparations, this hypothesis was confirmed. Drugs that cause few extrapyramidal side effects such as clozapine have the greatest affinity for muscarinic receptors, similar to that of classical anticholinergic agents (Snyder et al. 1974). In contrast, drugs such as haloperidol and fluphenazine, whose frequency of extrapyramidal effects are greater, have a much lower affinity for the muscarinic receptors. According to this hypothesis, when given at therapeutic antischizophrenic doses, all neuroleptics produce a dopamine receptor blockade and thus they all have about the same tendency to elicit extrapyramidal side effects. Simultaneous blockade of acetylcholine receptors by drugs such as clozapine or thioridazine antagonizes the extrapyramidal side effects. Because of their negligible anticholinergic activity at normal doses, drugs such as haloperidol elicit many more extrapyramidal side effects. Screening of potentially useful antipsychotic drugs for muscarinic receptor affinity may thus provide a simple *in vitro* predictor of their capacity to induce extrapyramidal side effects.

A similar explanation has been proposed to explain the varying propensity of neuroleptics to produce autonomic sympatholytic effects such as sedation and orthostatic hypotension. In this case, blocking the alpha-noradrenergic receptor appears to be the culprit. Neuroleptic affinity for alpha-noradrenergic receptors was studied by looking at their ability to compete with the binding of [^{3}H]WB4101, a potent alpha-antagonist (Peroutka et al. 1977). Neuroleptics, as a group, have high affinities for alpha receptors, within the same range as the affinities of neuroleptics for dopamine receptors. However, there is no correlation between an individual drug's affinity for alpha receptors compared to its affinity for dopamine receptors. Thus, a drug such as droperidol is potent both at alpha and dopamine receptors, while a drug such as spiroperidol is much more potent at dopamine than at alpha receptors. As an index of their alpha receptor antagonism, neuroleptics are often screened for their ability to act as antagonists of the lethal effects of intravenously administered norepinephrine in rats (Janssen and Van Bever 1975). This fatal alpha-noradrenergic vasopressor activity of norepinephrine is blocked by classical alpha receptor antagonists. The pharmacological relevance of [^{3}H]WB4101 binding sites is attested by the high correlation between the potencies of drugs in competing for [^{3}H]WB4101 binding and their potencies in blocking norepinephrine toxicity (fig. 6.9). This correlation across all neuroleptics is highly selective, since there is no significant correlation between affinities for alpha receptor binding sites and neuroleptic potency as measured in any dopamine receptor blocking test, such as production of catalepsy or antagonism of amphetamine or apomorphine stereotypy.

Because therapeutic brain levels of neuroleptics may be expected to correspond to concentrations of the drugs that are required to obtain an optimal blockade of dopamine receptors, the clinical propensity of neuroleptics to block alpha receptors *in vivo* would then be related not to their absolute potencies as alpha blockers but to the ratio of the relative potencies as alpha antagonists and dopamine antagonists. Drugs with low ratios (higher affinity for alpha receptors than dopamine receptors), such as clozapine, would be anticipated to elicit a substantial amount of alpha-noradrenergic blockade at blood and brain levels of the drug required for adequate dopamine receptor blockade and thus cause sedation and orthostatic hypotension. By contrast, drugs with high ratios, such as haloperidol, with higher affinity for dopamine receptors than alpha receptors, would be employed clinically at the very low dose levels required to secure dopamine receptor blockade and so, in general, would be less likely to elicit side effects associated with alpha-adrenergic blockade. Thus, screening new antipsychotic agents

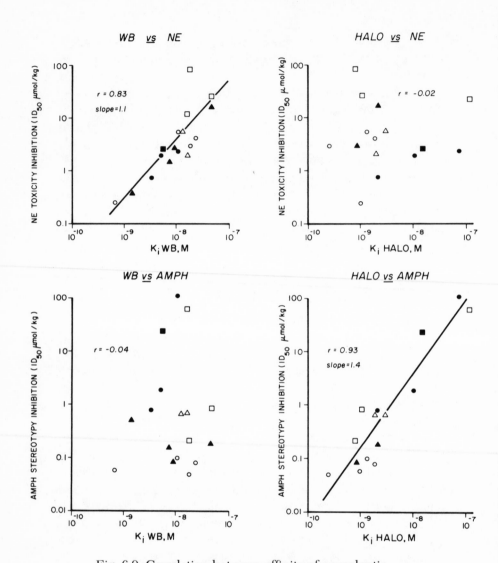

Fig. 6.9. Correlation between affinity of neuroleptic drugs for alpha-adrenergic receptors ([³H]WB-4101 binding) and dopamine receptors ([³H]haloperidol binding) and potency in antinorepinephrine and antiamphetamine tests. Neuroleptic drug classes: phenothiazines, ● = alkylamino, ■ = piperidine, ▲ = piperazine; ○ = butyrophenones; △ = thioxanthenes; □ − others. (From Peroutka et al. 1977.)

for affinity at alpha-adrenergic receptors gives insight into their propensity to cause side effects such as sedation and orthostatic hypotension.

Although more efficient drug screening has certainly been a beneficial spin-off from this research, this has not been its main goal. A "dopamine theory of schizophrenia" is certainly consistent with this work, although one should emphasize that the dopamine receptor mediation of the therapeutic action of neuroleptics does not necessarily mean that dopamine synapses are themselves disturbed in schizophrenia. The deficit may actually be elsewhere, and a normally functioning dopamine system may be merely a requirement for its manifestations. If indeed dopamine systems are abnormal in schizophrenia, there are several possible sites for the abnormalities. The evidence to date suggests a functional excess in dopaminergic activity that could result from too much dopamine being released, a decreased reuptake of dopamine, a decrease in enzymatic breakdown of dopamine, or perhaps an increased interaction of dopamine with its receptors. Such a receptor-mediated change could result either from an enhanced affinity of the receptors for dopamine or an increase in dopamine receptor numbers. We are at present attempting to test this hypothesis by measuring dopamine receptor binding in the brains of schizophrenics and patients who have died of nonneurological diseases.

To date, the evidence that an abnormality in the dopamine systems occurs in schizophrenics is circumstantial. As we learn more about neuronal functions and neurotransmitter receptors in the brain and the possible perturbations that may occur, we should be able to cast more light on the biochemistry of schizophrenia.

DISCUSSION

You imply that we may be able to find a drug that separates the main effects of antischizophrenic drugs from the side effects. Could you say more about this?

The one mechanism that we do know whereby we get antischizophrenic effect is by blocking the dopamine receptor, and of course there are many drugs on the market which do this. Now we know that at least in some parts of the brain there are relative antagonisms between gamma aminobutyric acid (GABA) activity and dopamine. In fact, there are specific GABA pathways that go from the corpus striatum down to the substantia nigra and inhibit dopamine neuronal firing. So if you mimic GABA, you would have a drug that would stop dopamine neurons from firing and that might be of interest. Of course, a drug that mimics GABA will act at GABA synapses all over the brain. While only one per cent of the synapses in the brain use dopamine as their transmitter, thirty to fifty percent use GABA; thus, GABA drugs may have many effects, and it is hard to say what those would turn out to be. But that is one approach that is being explored. The psychopharmacologic problem is to sort out desired effects without creating new side effects. This, I think, is a real frontier in psychopharmacology research.

Do you think it is still a good guess that there is a dopamine biochemical etiology for schizophrenia?

Certainly one might speculate that the lesion in schizophrenia is excess of dopamine, too many dopamine neurons, too much release of dopamine, too much synthesis of dopamine, too little metabolic degradation or an excess number of dopamine receptors, and so on, all in some specific part of the brain. That is possible. Of course, just because you can titrate schizophrenic symptoms up or down by titrating dopamine does not mean that dopamine is the locus of the disease. The basic biochemical mechanism could be several steps removed, just as aspirin, by inhibiting prostaglandin synthesis, presumably reduces fever. The fever was not caused in a fundamental sense by the prostaglandins; they were just a link along the way.

There seems to be a relation between the anticholinergic potency of drugs and their clinical potency. Is this a central phenomenon or an absorption phenomenon?

It is not related to absorption because that relation can be observed *in vitro*. That is, the more potent antidopamine drugs *in vitro* have less potent anticholinergic effects. What has happened is that the drugs that we use have been screened to eliminate anticholinergic activity, and those are the drugs that we use clinically.

Is there some relation between alpha-adrenergic propensity and hypotension?

The work on the alpha-adrenergic receptor is very recent, so we have not gone into a great detail about the different drugs. Haloperidol is a very potent alpha-adrenergic blocker. However, it is so potent clinically that we use it at very low doses. At the doses that are used I do not know how much central alpha-adrenergic blockade we get. Haloperidol is, however, very lipid soluble, so that its partitioning between brain and periphery may be much greater than for other neuroleptics. I would speculate that you may obtain high brain levels with relatively low levels in the periphery, and of course the periphery is where you have your hypotension.

REFERENCES

Angrist, B., G. Sathanthan, and S. Gershon. 1973. Behavioral effects of L-dopa in schizophrenic patients. *Psychopharmacologia* 31:1–12.

Bunney, B. S., J. R. Walters, R. H. Roth, and G. K. Aghajanian. 1973. Dopaminergic neurons, effect of antipsychotic drugs and amphetamine on single cell activity. *Journal of Pharmacology and Experimental Therapeutics* 185:560–571.

Burt, D. R., I Creese, and S. H. Snyder. 1976a. Binding interactions of LSD and related agents with dopamine receptors in the brain. *Molecular Pharmacology* 12:631–638.

_____. 1976b. Characteristics of [^{3}H]haloperidol and [^{3}H]dopamine binding associated with dopamine receptors in calf brain membranes. *Molecular Pharmacology* 12:800–812.

_____. 1977. Antischizophrenic drugs: chronic treatment elevates dopamine receptor binding in the brain. *Science* 196:326–328.

_____. Burt, D. R., S. Enna, I. Creese, and S. H. Snyder. 1975. Dopamine receptor binding in the corpus striatum of mammalian brain. *Proceedings of the National Academy of Sciences of the United States of America* 172:4655–4659.

Carlsson, A., and J. Lindqvist. 1963. Effects of chlorpromazine and haloperidol on the formation of 3-methoxytyramine and normetanephrine in mouse brain. *Acta Pharmacologica and Toxicologia* 20:140–144.

Connell, P. H. 1958. *Amphetamine psychosis*. London: Chapman and Hall.

Creese, I., D. R. Burt, and S. H. Snyder. 1975. Dopamine receptor binding: differentiation of agonist and antagonist states with [^{3}H]dopamine and [^{3}H]haloperidol. *Life Science* 17:993–1002.

_____. 1976a. Dopamine receptor binding predicts clinical and pharmacological potencies of antischizophrenic drugs. *Science* 192:481–483.

_____. 1976b. Dopamine receptors and average clinical doses. *Science* 194:546.

_____. 1977. Dopamine receptor binding enhancement accompanies lesion-induced behavioral supersensitivity. *Science* 197:596–598.

Creese, I., R. Schneider, and S. H. Snyder. 1977. [^{3}H]Spiroperidol labels brain and pituitary dopamine receptors. *European Journal of Pharmacology* 46:377–381.

Friedhoff, A. J., and E. Van Winkle. 1963. 3,4-dimethoxyphenylethylamine and other amines in the urine of schizophrenic patients. *Nature* 199:203–204.

Iversen, L. L., M. A. Rogawski, and R. J. Miller. 1976. Comparison of the effects of neuroleptic drugs on pre- and postsynaptic dopaminergic mechanisms in the rat striatum. *Molecular Pharmacology* 12:251–262.

Janowsky, D. S., M. K. El-Yousef, J. M. Davis, and H. J. Sekerka. 1973. Provocation of schizophrenic symptoms by intravenous administration of methylphenidate. *Archives of General Psychiatry* 28:185–191.

Janssen, P. A. J., and W. F. Van Bever. 1975. Advances in the search for improved neuroleptic drugs. In *Current developments in psychopharmacology,* vol. 2, ed. W. B. Essman and L. Valzelli. New York: Spectrum.

Kebabian, J. W., G. L. Petzold, and P. Greengard. 1972. Dopamine-sensitive adenylate cyclase in caudate nucleus of rat brain and its similarity to the "dopamine receptor." *Proceedings of the National Academy of Sciences of the United States of America* 69:2145–2149.

Kety, S. S. 1959. Biochemical theories of schizophrenia. *Science* 129:1528–1532.

Klawans, H. L. 1973. The pharmacology of tardive dyskinesia. *American Journal of Psychiatry* 130:82–86.

Klein, D. F., and J. M. Davis. 1969. *Diagnosis and treatment of psychiatric disorders.* Baltimore: Williams and Wilkins.

Kobayashi, R. M. 1977. Drug therapy of tardive dyskinesia. *New England Journal of Medicine* 296:257–260.

Peroutka, S. J., D. C. U'Prichard, D. A. Greenberg, and S. H. Snyder. 1977. Neuroleptic drug interactions with norepinephrine α-receptor binding sites in rat brain. *Neuropharmacology,* 16:549–556.

Perry, T., S. Hansen, and L. MacDougall. 1967. Identity and significance of some pink spots in schizophrenia and other conditions. *Nature* 214:484–485.

Pieri, L., M. Pieri, and W. Haefely. 1974. LSD as an agonist of dopamine receptors in the striatum. *Nature* 252:556–588.

Randrup, A., and I. Munkvad. 1970. Biochemical, anatomical and psychological investigations of stereotyped behavior induced by amphetamines. In *Amphetamines and related compounds,* ed. E. Costa and S. Garattini. New York: Raven Press.

Seeman, P., M. Chau-Wong, J. Tedesco, and K. Wong. 1975. Brain receptors for antipsychotic drugs and dopamine: direct binding assays. *Proceedings of the National Academy of Sciences of the United States of America* 72:4376–4380.

Siegel, M., and H. Tefft. 1971. "Pink spot" and its components in normal and schizophrenic urine. *Journal of Nervous Mental Disorders* 152:412–426.

Snyder, S. H. 1975a. Neurotransmitter and drug receptors in the brain. *Biochemical Pharmacology* 24:1371–1374.

————. 1975b. Opiate receptor in normal and drug altered brain function. *Nature* 257:185–189.

Snyder, S. H., S. P. Banerjee, H. I. Yamamura, and D. A. Greenberg. 1974. Drugs, neurotransmitters and schizophrenia. *Science* 184:1243–1253.

Snyder, S. H., I. Creese, and D. R. Burt. 1975. The brain's dopamine receptor: labeling with [³H]dopamine and [³H]haloperidol. *Psychopharmacology Communications* 1:663–673.

Tarsy, D., and R. J. Baldessarini. 1974. Behavioral supersensitivity to apomorphine following chronic treatment with drugs which interfere with the synaptic function of catecholamines. *Neuropharmacology* 13:927–940.

Ungerstedt, U. 1971. Postsynaptic supersensitivity after 6-hydroxydopamine induced degeneration of the nigrostriatal dopamine system. *Acta Physiologica Scandinavica* (supplement) 367:69–93.

Voith, K., and J. R. Cummings. 1976. Behavioral studies on the enantiomers of butaclamol demonstrating absolute optical specificity for neuroleptic activity. *Canadian Journal of Physiology* 54:551–560.

Von Hungen, K., S. Roberts, and D. F. Hill. 1975. Interactions between lysergic acid diethylamide and dopamine-sensitive adenylate cyclase systems in rat brain. *Brain Research* 94:57–66.

7

Psychopharmacology

LEO HOLLISTER

After almost a quarter of a century of experience, one can say with reasonable confidence that antipsychotic drugs are the sheet anchor of treatment for schizophrenia. The efficacy of antipsychotic drugs has been easy to prove in controlled clinical trials, something not so easily done with alternative treatments. One could almost state categorically that no other treatment has been proven as effective in schizophrenia. However, while these drugs control the symptoms of schizophrenia, they do not cure the disorder. We have many patients who are better, but none who are well. Some critics have denigrated symptomatic control by referring to these drugs as chemical straitjackets. More likely these drugs have functioned as liberating agents, making a more nearly normal life possible for many schizophrenics who might have been hospitalized for a lifetime. The number of hospitalized patients with schizophrenia has declined steadily since the advent of drugs, especially so in the past few years. Of course many other factors have decreased the need for hospital care; yet reductions of hospitalized patients to twenty-five percent (a frequent figure) of what had been the case ten to fifteen years ago would hardly have been possible without drugs. Furthermore, symptomatic control does not mean that the drugs are not acting on some basic pathogenetic process involved in schizophrenia. It simply means that they are not acting on all such processes. Drug treatment for schizophrenia compares reasonably well with that for congestive heart failure. We must never remain content with the drugs that we have.

A corollary to this appraisal of drug treatment is that we should not neglect other treatments that help the schizophrenic patient. Many of the basic amenities of life, assumed by all of us to be rights, are considered to be privileges, or even worse, to be treatment for schizophrenics. The word "therapy" has been used for every banal activity of life. Surely, a humane approach to the victims of this disorder is their right, and not something conferred by a "therapist." Despite the difficulty in proving the efficacy of treatments other than drugs, empirically derived experience suggests that some therapies may help. I am personally convinced that insight psychotherapy, either attempted as individual or as group psychotherapy, is useless for the schizophrenic. On the other hand, group psychotherapy aimed at providing guides to resocialization, helping the patient function unobtrusively in society, and establishing some sort of social life is certainly worthwhile. Occupational therapy may be helpful for patients with less severe emotional disorders but is useless for schizophrenics. What they need is true vocational training, so that they can perform useful, simple jobs that will provide for their partial support and provide them the dignity that comes from honest work. In short, the schizophrenic might best be viewed as a handicapped individual whose residual assets must be utilized. In this way, the symptomatic control from drug treatment can be extended to enrich the lives of patients.

Let us consider when antipsychotic drugs should not be used. They are not indicated for most acute brain syndromes, especially those associated with acute reactions to social drugs, such as cannabis or hallucinogens, or withdrawal from abused drugs, such as alcohol or opiates. Available evidence suggests that the treatment is worse than the illness. Antipsychotic drugs are not only less effective than conventional sedatives but may actually be harmful. The acute brain syndrome seen in desperately ill patients placed in the unfamiliar and weird surroundings of an explosive medical technology is an exception. Small doses of antipsychotic drugs, notably haloperidol but very likely others of high potency and specificity, ameliorate the "intensive-care unit psychosis." Antipsychotic drugs are not indicated for minor disorders such as simple anxiety, despite their promotion for such use based on their low potential for abuse. Abuse of conventional anti-anxiety drugs used under medical supervision is uncommon. Unwarranted fears should not lead to unjustified treatments. These drugs are not indicated for patients who have, or who may have, endogenous depressions. Tricyclic antidepressants are clearly the drugs of choice for this disorder. Antipsychotics may make matters worse, if only by delaying effective treatment.

Antipsychotic drugs are useful in a number of disorders. First, they are the basic treatment of *schizophrenia*. Even the last bastions of resistance, the psychoanalytic institutes, now use drugs for schizophrenics. The extensive literature of evaluative trials, constituting the most massive scientific overkill in all clinical pharmacology, has demonstrated the value of antipsychotic drugs in all forms of schizophrenia, at all ages, at all stages of illness, and in all parts of the world. Alas, not in all patients, at least to any meaningful degree.

Given that drugs are a primary treatment, does this necessarily mean that they should be given indiscriminately to all schizophrenic patients? Some patients have rather good premorbid adjustments and their psychosis has relatively clear precipitants. Such patients have been termed as having "reactive" schizophrenia, or in European literature, schizophreniform psychoses. Drugs may be useful during the acute episode but are probably not required for maintenance after its resolution. Another group of patients for whom drug therapy might be questioned are those with exceedingly chronic schizophrenia and long-term hospitalization. Often such patients show only meaningless improvement from drug therapy, which is more often given for the benefit of the hospital staff than for the benefit of the patient. The need of such patients for drug treatment has been questioned, especially since this group seems most vulnerable to tardive dyskinesia. This latter complication should lead to the most conservative use of these drugs. Unfortunately, a current trend is in the opposite direction. Even patients with acute schizophrenia, where drugs are most clearly indicated, may be overtreated in the zeal to reduce hospital stay or even to avoid hospitalization. Nor do all chronically psychotic patients require large doses of these drugs or prolonged, uninterrupted treatment. The risks for some may outweigh the benefits.

Second, the preponderance of evidence suggests that antipsychotic drugs are the preferred treatment for *schizoaffective disorders*. Some patients respond to lithium alone and some respond better to combined treatment.

Third, acute manic states associated with *manic-depressive disorder* often require antipsychotic drugs for effective management. Lithium is the primary treatment, but because of its slow onset of action, concurrent use of an antipsychotic may be required for a period of several days.

Fourth, antipsychotic drugs have been used to treat *depression*. Most studies comparing these drugs with tricyclics in heterogeneous groups of depressed patients have failed to show much difference in response, but use of these drugs remains controversial. Arguments against their use can be stated as follows: they will probably make truly endogenous depressions worse; they are not necessarily more effective than placebo, antianxiety drugs, or the sedative tricyclic antidepressants in the mixed anxiety–depression syndrome so often associated with reactive depressions; the risk of tardive dyskinesias is too great under these conditions. Some patients undoubtedly are helped more by these drugs than by any other type, but antipsychotic drugs are not a preferred treatment.

Fifth, *Gilles de la Tourette Syndrome* is a rare disorder (there may be only a few hundred such patients in the entire United States) that responds to antipsychotic drugs. Haloperidol, the only drug adequately studied, is preferred, although benefit may not be unique to this drug. The unpredictable barking tic and outbursts of foul language these patients suffer are socially disabling, and drug treatment is clearly warranted.

And finally, although best results in true organic brain syndromes of *senile* or *arteriosclerotic brain disease* have been obtained from antipsychotics, the goals of treatment are limited.

All antipsychotic drugs share two novel pharmacological actions that were unknown prior to their advent: the ability to ameliorate the course of schizophrenia and the ability to evoke in many patients extrapyramidal syndromes of various types, including one that strongly mimics naturally occurring Parkinson's disease. For a long time it was uncertain why these two unusual and seemingly unrelated effects should be linked. Now it appears that both are mediated through the same biochemical mechanism, decreased dopaminergic transmission in those pathways in the brain that use this neurotransmitter. The fact that antipsychotic drugs block postsynaptic dopamine receptors, as well as other evidence based largely on clinical observations and biochemical studies, had led to the popular "dopamine hypothesis" of schizophrenia. While this hypothesis has been of heuristic value, it is quite clear that overactivity of dopaminergic systems accounts for only a part of the schizophrenic disorder.

Electrophysiologic studies indicate that these drugs affect the function of the three major integrating systems of the brain, the reticular activating system, the limbic system, and the hypothalamus. One might speculate that they could reduce extraneous or distracting sensory information, reduce the affective charge of all sensations, and reduce the somatic responses to them. Much more needs to be known about the actions of the drugs and the pathogenetic mechanism of schizophrenia. All of us are desperately looking for new leads.

About twenty drugs are marketed in the United States as antipsychotics. Phenothiazine derivatives are both the most numerous and still the most widely used. Three chemical subfamilies can be distinguished, based on differences in the side-chain. The aliphatic series and the piperidine series of compounds are generally regarded as low potency compounds, the daily therapeutic doses being measured in hundreds of milligrams; the piperazine series are high potency compounds, with daily doses measured in tens of milligrams.

The modification in the ring of the thioxanthenes tends to make for a generally less potent group of compounds than for the phenothiazines. Such seems to be the case for chlorprothixene, the thioxanthene homologue of chlorpromazine. The slight loss of potency from the ring structure can be compensated for by the choice of ring substituents and side-chains. The dimethylsulfonamide ring substituent and piperazine side-chain of thiothixene make it a fairly potent drug. Potency should never be confused with efficacy, however, which is roughly the same overall among these drugs. The separation of antipsychotic effects from other pharmacological actions of these drugs, such as sedation or alpha-adrenergic blockade, may reduce certain side effects while increasing others, such as extrapyramidal motor reactions. The

French phrase for such a drug is *neuroleptique incisif,* the English equivalent being "a more specific antipsychotic drug."

Although many butyrophenone structures are possible, haloperidol is the only one currently marketed in the United States. Molindone and loxapine, two new entries into the market, are effective antipsychotic drugs, but it remains to be seen whether they have any special advantage over previous drugs other than the dubious one of representing a different chemical structure.

A completely rational choice between antipsychotic drugs cannot currently be made for individual patients. After devoting more than ten years to trying to find specific indications for various antipsychotic drugs, I have finally concluded that it cannot be done on the basis of presenting symptoms and signs of schizophrenia. One of the most rational ways to narrow the choice of antipsychotics would be to master one of each of the three types of phenothiazines and one of each of the remaining chemical classes of drugs. A possible selection, based on drugs currently available in the United States, is as follows:

Phenothiazines
 Aliphatic: chlorpromazine
 Piperidine: thioridazine
 Piperazine: fluphenazine
Thioxanthenes: thiothixene
Butyrophenones: haloperidol
Dibenzoxazepines: loxapine
Indolics: molindone

A basic assumption in making these choices is that differences within a chemical class are less than differences between classes, thus allowing the choice of only a single drug for each class. The assumption is also made that the puzzling differences between the responses of individual patients to different drugs (a clinical phenomenon that was recognized as soon as more than one drug became available) are largely due to differences in the patient's metabolic handling of the drug, making chemical distinctions important. Overriding all other considerations is the patient's past history of response to a drug, if that information is available.

Most of what we know of the pharmacokinetics of antipsychotics—that is, the fate of these drugs in the body—is derived from studies on chlorpromazine. This drug has been most widely studied not only because it is the prototype but also because it is given in relatively high doses, so that greater quantities of drug and its metabolites can be measured. Nevertheless, technical problems in measuring these are formidable. Chlorpromazine may have the most extensive metabolism of any psychoactive drug. As many as 160 possible metabolites have been posited, most of which are inactive. Very little drug is excreted unchanged in urine, most appearing as glucuronide metabolites. Absorption of orally administered chlorpromazine is erratic. Anything that delays absorption, whether it be the type of pharmaceutical preparation or the presence of other drugs that slow gastrointestinal motility, diminishes the amount of unchanged drug reaching the circulation. The drug may be metabolized both in the gut as well as by its first passage through the liver. Chlorpromazine is both highly protein-bound and highly lipid soluble, with a large apparent volume of distribution. These factors allow accumulation of the drug.

One might imagine the body to be a huge sponge that must be saturated. To do this expeditiously, large initial doses may be required. Once the sponge is saturated, one needs only to replace what is lost (by metabolism in this case), a generally smaller amount. When the drug is discontinued, therapeutic effects may persist for variable periods, as the sponge takes a while to dry out (or in this case, for all drug to be eliminated). The length of these periods would depend on the amount of drug accumulated and its rate of elimination in a particular patient.

Intramuscularly administered drug, which bypasses the gut and the liver, reaches the circulation more readily and is far more available to the brain. In the case of chlorpromazine, the potency ratio to oral doses may be about four to one. The higher potency of drugs such as haloperidol and fluphenazine may be due to less extensive metabolism, and consequently this potency ratio may differ. Almost anything we say about the pharmacokinetics of these drugs is based on extrapolations, which may not be correct, from chlorpromazine.

Few drugs have such great therapeutic margins and such a

wide range of therapeutic doses as do antipsychotic drugs. Those shown in table 7.1 are only rough guides, somewhat reflecting current practice towards using higher doses. It remains to be seen whether this trend is justified. The old idea of a "digitalizing" dose has been revived for antipsychotic drugs, resulting in doses of 50 to 100 mg of fluphenazine in rapid increments. It is now known, of course, that the digitalis effect is a graded phenomenon and not an all-or-none effect. As it seems almost certain that the same principle applies to antipsychotics, one might question the risk of overtreating many patients for the somewhat dubious gain of shortening hospitalization for a few. We tend to

Table 7.1. Dosage relationships among antipsychotic drugs.

Generic name	Relative potency	Range of total daily dose (mg)	
		Outpatient	Inpatient
Phenothiazines			
Aliphatic			
chlorpromazine	100	50–400	200–1600
Piperidine			
thioridazine	100	50–400	200–800
mesoridazine	50	25–200	100–400
piperacetazine	10	10–40	20–160
Piperazine			
carphenazine	25	50–150	75–400
acetophenazine	20	40–80	60–100
prochlorperazine	15	20–60	60–200
perphenazine	10	8–24	12–64
butaperazine	10	10–30	10–100
trifluoperazine	5	4–10	10–60
fluphenazine	2	1–5	2–60
Thioxanthene			
thiothixene	5	6–30	10–120
Butyrophenones			
haloperidol	2	2–6	4–100
Dibenzoxazepines			
loxapine	10	15–60	40–160
Indolics			
molindone	10	15–60	40–225

hurry too much in treating schizophrenics, where it generally does not much matter, and too little in treating depressives, where it does.

The possibility of monitoring doses of antipsychotics by measuring plasma levels of the drug seems to be quite remote. For the moment the clinician might surmise that an inadequate dose of drug has been delivered in the absence of either an improved mental state or an extrapyramidal reaction. These are the two novel pharmacological actions of these drugs, each of which bears somewhat on the other. If neither outcome is evident, then the optimal dose has not been attained. However, exploration of the upper limits of effective dose should be based on other considerations. Obviously, routine use of an antiparkinson drug at the onset of treatment may rob the clinician of one of these two clinical criteria for assessing the adequacy of dose.

One of the more common errors in drug prescription found in a large mental hospital was excessively low doses. One should not be so afraid of doing harm that one does no good. Other errors commonly encountered were excessive use of antiparkinson medication and the use of irrational combinations of drugs, including the use of antidepressants for schizophrenics. Nothing will substitute for careful thought if drugs are to be used well; treatment should never, repeat never, become routine.

When starting treatment, divided doses are usually given—that is, smaller quantities are given at more frequent intervals than would be the case later in the treatment. These divided doses minimize the initial impact of many of the unwanted pharmacological effects (sedation and adrenergic blocking activity) and allow better titration of dose. Unfortunately, this practice, eminently sensible in initiating treatment, is seldom changed later in the treatment, and patients may stay on divided doses for years. As these drugs are intrinsically long-acting, no pharmacokinetic basis for divided doses obtains. Once a patient reaches a satisfactory daily maintenance dose, it is feasible to reduce the frequency. Many clinicians aim for a single daily dose to be given just before retiring and, even when they use divided doses, tend to give the major dose of the day at this time. Two advantages accrue. The patient sleeps when he should, not because he is oversedated during the day. Second, he is less likely to suffer disabling extrapyramidal symptoms if the major impact of the drug occurs while he is sleeping. For reasons still not clear, manifestations of Parkinson's disease are ameliorated by sleep.

The procedure for reducing doses may vary. Some prefer to eliminate the morning dose first, consolidating it with one given later in the day and then progressively doing the same to noon and afternoon doses. If very large amounts of drug are required for maintenance treatment, one may still prefer to divide the total daily dose, giving perhaps one-third in the late afternoon and the rest before bedtime. In most cases, however, the goal of a single daily maintenance dose can be attained. Many drugs are now available in larger single-dose units to meet the growing acceptance of the single daily dose.

As a rule, schizophrenic patients should be placed on maintenance doses that are as low as possible while retaining therapeutic gains. Dosage should be reduced gradually to avoid a sudden recrudescence of symptoms. The minimal dose at which the patient functions best is preferred. Reduction of doses for maintenance treatment is of considerable importance. My own feeling is that many instances of so-called postschizophrenic depression are due to overtreatment with antipsychotic drugs. As one becomes more "normal," these drugs become more noxious; one might even postulate biochemical reasons why an excess of drug might evoke depression. This explanation is more acceptable to me than the idea that the depression is a reaction to the realization that one is schizophrenic.

The observance of "drug holidays" is another way in which the total exposure of patients to drugs may be reduced. Such an approach is completely empirical, as it is impossible to predict in advance which patient will tolerate a drug holiday of any substantial period of time. Unless someone is around to watch the patient carefully for signs of relapse, so that treatment may be resumed immediately, this approach is neither feasible nor fair to the patient. Nor has it been shown that exposure to drugs can be reduced further by this approach than by trying assiduously to find the least possible maintenance dose.

Many patients take their own drug holidays, either by discontinuing the drug altogether or by taking less than prescribed.

Thirty-nine of eighty-five chronic schizophrenic patients took less drug than prescribed when followed over a two-year period. The major reason proposed for discontinuation was the unpleasant effect of a subtle akathisia. Actually, this rate of noncompliance is not much different from that of patients taking antihypertensive drugs or those on prophylactic regimens of antituberculosis drugs.

Assuming that one has found the minimal maintenance dose, the patient should be cautioned to continue medication even though he feels well and should be reassured about fears of becoming addicted. He should be cautioned about possible drowsiness and interference with skilled movements and warned against the concomitant use of alcoholic beverages. The patient's family should have the same instruction. Information should be provided to the family physician and pharmacist. An uninterrupted supply of medication should be assured. The ever-increasing number of patients discharged from hospitals on antipsychotic drugs poses a special challenge to followup clinics.

Long-acting depot preparations have been a boon to maintenance therapy, especially when patients are unreliable about taking medication. Several studies prove a decreased rate of relapse among patients so maintained, as contrasted with those taking daily oral medication.

No proof that I know of substantiates the combination of any antipsychotic drugs. Uniformly, combinations have not been more effective than adequate use of the single most appropriate drug. Antiparkinson drugs are most often combined with antipsychotics, and when done to treat established drug-induced extrapyramidal reactions, this combination is good treatment. Routine use of antiparkinson drugs prior to development of an extrapyramidal reaction is seldom indicated, representing a major source of drug overuse.

A combination of a tricyclic antidepressant and an antipsychotic may be justified when the diagnosis is uncertain between a schizoaffective disorder with depression or an endogenous depression with psychotic manifestations. The tricyclic is generally useless simply for treating the emotional withdrawal and motor retardation of the schizophrenic. When such a combination is needed, it would seem well to use perphenazine and amitriptyline, which has been widely used clinically with little difficulty. Extemporaneous combinations, with doses adjusted flexibly, would be preferred.

Some manic patients require antipsychotic drugs during initial treatment with lithium, as the latter drug alone may not curb severe mania. Whether or not some schizophrenic patients can benefit from the addition of lithium to treatment remains to be determined. One is tempted to regard such responses as indicating a misdiagnosis of schizophrenia in a manic patient.

Some patients still complain of anxiety and insomnia, despite large doses of antipsychotics given at night. Auxiliary use of one of the benzodiazepines may be rational for treating these symptoms and is preferable to increasing the dose of antipsychotic.

Many older side effects that used to be of much concern, such as agranulocytosis and cholestatic jaundice, are now rarely encountered. Possibly this shift is due to the increasing use of more potent drugs, which are seldom associated with these complications. Baseline laboratory tests are obligatory on all patients, with possibly a repeat in the first few weeks of treatment; after that, they may be obtained at much longer intervals or only as needed.

The side effect of the Parkinsonian syndrome, now known to be inextricably tied to the antipsychotic action, is easily managed by antiparkinsonian drugs. In many instances, it appears to be self-limiting, so that auxiliary treatment for more than a few weeks is unnecessary. Acute dystonic reactions early in treatment and akathisia are other variants of this syndrome.

Tardive dyskinesias have been of increasing concern, their frequency of occurrence almost depending on how closely one looks for the complication. They need not be in old patients (some have been observed in children) nor in patients under long treatment (some develop within weeks). The fact that they may occur in nonpsychotic patients treated with antipsychotic drugs is warning enough against using these drugs for trivial indications. The basic mechanism proposed for the development of this syndrome is the development of dopaminergic hyperactivity in the striato-nigral system, with a relative reduction in cholinergic function. Such a formulation explains several clinical phenomena. (1) Most, if not all, cases of tardive dyskinesia are preceded by the Parkinsonian syndrome, and occasionally one sees mixed syndromes. (2) Anticholinergic drugs are not only ineffective but often unmask a latent dyskinesia. (3) Augmenting doses of antipsychotic drugs, either by using more of the same or adding another, often ameliorate the picture, at least temporarily. (4) Sudden withdrawal from an antipsychotic drug may exacerbate a latent syndrome. (5) Levodopa makes it worse and physostigmine may briefly ameliorate it.

Treatment of tardive dyskinesia, either by attempting to decrease dopaminergic activity or by increasing cholinergic activity, has generally been disappointing. Early recognition of the syndrome and gradual reduction in doses of the antipsychotic drug may be the best strategy. The choice may be hard: one must balance control of schizophrenia against increasing the abnormal movements.

The phenomenon of sudden, unexpected, and unexplained death in otherwise healthy individuals treated with antipsychotics has been a matter of some controversy for many years. It is fortunately a rare event, superimposed upon a "normal" background of such deaths. Thus, one can never be sure that these deaths are drug-related. Those of us who are convinced that they *are* drug-related believe that one should change treatment if one sees drug-induced changes in ventricular repolarization on the electrocardiogram and that caution is needed in the patient with preexisting intraventricular block or premature ventricular contractions. A history of brief syncopal attacks during established treatment may be a warning of self-limited episodes of ventricular tachyarrhythmia. Other than this, one cannot do much to prevent these disasters.

To summarize these general principles of treatment: One should use antipsychotic drugs primarily to treat schizophrenia. They are too potent to use for trivial purposes or where other, safer, and often cheaper drugs are suitable. Their use does not preclude other therapeutic approaches but rather makes these approaches more fruitful.

The dose should be tailored to the needs of the individual patient. Interpatient variability in dose requirements has long been noted. Recently, measurements of plasma concentrations of drugs confirm this degree of variability. Individualization of doses may be based on two clinical criteria: improvement of schizophrenia or development of extrapyramidal motor reactions. Reducing maintenance doses of drug is often overlooked, but this step may be essential if some complications of treatment are to be avoided.

Dosage schedules do not have to fit the usual equally divided, several-times-a-day pattern. These are long-acting drugs and therefore do not require frequent doses. Often a once-daily dosage is adequate; even when doses are divided, they need not be equally divided.

Duration of drug treatment should be determined by clinical judgment. It may be briefly interrupted on weekends or during acute illnesses, but prolonged drug holidays may be less effective in reducing total exposure to the drug than simple reduction in maintenance dosage schedules.

Finally, the form in which the dose is given may be important. Kinetic studies indicate that slow absorption of the drug through the gut decreases bioavailability. Intramuscular doses are more efficient, although the potency ratio for some of the newer, "low-dose" drugs is unknown. Long-acting depot forms may be suitable for maintenance when compliance is a problem.

DISCUSSION

The maintenance level of antipsychotic medication is often difficult for clinicians to decide upon. Can you give any guidelines concerning maintenance dose?

Maintenance doses of antipsychotics can only be arrived at by titration of the needs of each individual patient. They should be as low as possible to maintain the maximal amount of remission, after an initial "saturation" dose. Thus, a maintenance dose may be a fraction of the maximal therapeutic dose used during the initiation of treatment. Sometimes the required maintenance dose falls into a narrow range. More often, as exemplified by successful drug holidays, the amount of drug in the body required for therapeutic effect may persist for periods without additional doses.

What is your practice with patients who are having their first psychotic episode? Do you keep all such patients on antipsychotics for a prolonged period?

Probably all patients who have an initial episode of schizophrenia should be treated with antipsychotic drugs, although a substantial number may remit without them. These cases may represent misdiagnoses or may represent the so-called "reactive" type of schizophrenia, which may be somewhat self-limited. Drug treatment may reduce the length of the episode. When it is possible to recognize such patients clearly, drug treatment may be stopped within a few weeks after remission; often the patient requests it or complains of feeling depressed from the drug.

The difficulty arises with the patient who fits more into the category of "process" schizophrenia, with a poor premorbid adjustment and an insidious onset. Such patients often fall short of complete remission on drug treatment. Maintenance doses should be gradually reduced and, unless the patient shows clear signs of relapse, a drug holiday may be tried if the patient can be observed for signs of relapse by someone responsible for his welfare and if the treatment can be resumed quickly if necessary. Even here, one is sometimes loath to stop drugs entirely, especially if the patient is working or has been able to return to school or has devised a satisfactory independent living arrangement. One tends to follow the old baseball adage: "Don't break up a winning combination."

Would you advocate taking the risks of long-term side effects for all patients with process schizophrenia, including those who would have done well off medication?

A number of studies of discontinuation of treatment in chronically maintained schizophrenics show that the majority will remain free of signs of obvious relapse for as long as four months. The catch is that there is absolutely no way to predict which patients can successfully go without drugs. If we could, drug holidays would be safe and reasonable. But as it is, the routine prescription of drug holidays will lead to relapse in a sizeable number of patients, potentially rehospitalizing them and breaking up a tenuous but nonetheless adequate social adjustment. If long-term complications can be prevented by reducing the patient's total exposure to the drug, then it makes equally good sense to use well titrated minimal maintenance doses without interruption. Drug holidays are often begun when the patient is on high maintenance doses, and when the patient has relapsed, as will almost inevitably be the case, high doses may be required for retreatment. It is a matter of clinical judgment, but I prefer the minimal maintenance procedure over the drug holiday. Proof about which is more effective in preventing tardive dyskinesia is totally lacking.

Would you comment on the problem of predicting outcome?

Predicting outcome for individual patients has been very difficult, even though one can make estimates for groups of patients. The difficulty is that we may set our treatment goals too high. Many years ago, during one of the Veterans' Administration cooperative studies, we investigated a group of patients whose average hospitalization exceeded eight years. Yet when we asked for a prognosis in order to determine their future needs for hospitalization, the mean estimate was an additional eight months. Clearly, we must have such delusions to persuade ourselves that treating such difficult patients is worthwhile.

If we were to set realistic goals for treatment of schizophrenic patients, based on all our knowledge of the patient's deficits and assets, we might be better able to predict outcome. Duration of hospitalization per se is the weakest criterion, as this judgment is purely arbitrary, affected either by the views of the psychiatrist or the constraints of the law. We might try to predict how well the patient would be able to care for himself in some quasi-independent living arrangement, or whether or not he would be employable, or whether or not he would be able to establish some satisfying social life. To predict the outcome I would be more concerned about these matters than about how well he ranked on some rating scale of psychiatric symptoms and signs.

REFERENCES

Expectations
Hollister, L. E. 1975. Drugs for emotional disorders: current problems. *Journal of the American Medical Association* 234:942–947.
Hogarty, G. E., and S. C. Goldberg. 1973. Drugs and sociotherapy in the aftercare of schizophrenic patients. *Archives of General Psychiatry* 28:54–64.

Indications
Baldessarini, R. J., and J. F. Lipinski. 1973. Risks versus benefits of antipsychotic drugs. *New England Journal of Medicine* 289:427–428.
Prien, R. F., R. D. Gillis, and E. M. Caffey. 1973. Intermittent pharmacotherapy in chronic schizophrenia. *Hospital and Community Psychiatry* 24(5):317–322.

Mode of Action
Hollister, L. E. 1973. *Clinical use of psychotherapeutic drugs.* Springfield, Ill.: Charles C Thomas.

Choice of Drug
Hollister, L. E. 1970. Choice of antipsychotic drugs. *American Journal of Psychiatry* 127:186–190.
Hollister, L. E., J. E. Overall, I. Kimbell, and A. Pokorny. 1974. Specific indications for different classes of phenothiazines. *Archives of General Psychiatry* 30:94–99.

Pharmacokinetics

Janssen, P. A. J. 1976. Structure-activity relationships (SAR) and drug design as illustrated with neuroleptic agents. In *Antipsychotic drugs: pharmacodynamics and pharmacokinetics,* ed. G. Sedvall, B. Uvnas, and Y. Zotterman. Oxford: Pergamon Press.

Doses

Laska, E. E. V., J. Wanderling, G. Simpson, G. W. Logemann, and B. K. Shah. 1973. Patterns of psychotropic drug use for schizophrenia. *Diseases of the Nervous System* 34:294–305.

Maintenance Therapy

Crawford, R., and A. Forrest. 1974. Controlled trial of depot fluphenazine in outpatient schizophrenics. *British Journal of Psychiatry* 124:385–391.

Morgan, R., and J. Cheadle. 1974. Maintenance treatment of chronic schizohrenia with neuroleptic drugs. *Acta Psychiatrica Scandinavica* 50:78–85.

Side Effects

Gerlach, J., N. Reisby, and A. Randrup. 1974. Dopaminergic hypersensitivity and cholinergic hypofunction in the pathophysiology of tardive dyskinesia. *Psychopharmacologia* 34:21–35.

PART FOUR

Care and Treatment: The Human Dimension

8

The Patient
and the Community

JONATHAN F. BORUS AND ELAINE HATOW

Two major roles must be filled if we are to deal effectively with schizophrenic persons. The scientific investigator must attempt to provide useful data that will improve our understanding of the etiology and elaboration of the state, and the practitioner-healer must attempt to use available data to better care for the patient. The focus in this chapter will be on the caregiving role, specifically on what the psychiatric physician and his allies can do to alleviate the immense suffering, disruption, and expense that schizophrenia brings to the individual, his family, and the community.

Psychiatric practitioners must provide ongoing care for schizophrenic patients while acknowledging that we do not yet know the scientific etiology (or etiologies) of, and specific remedies for, this illness. As Osler pointed out to graduating medical students almost a century ago in *Aequanimitas* (1922), caregiving in the face of such uncertainty is a major part of a physician's role: "A distressing feature in the life you are about to enter, a feature which will press hardly upon the finer spirits among you and ruffle their equanimity, is the uncertainty which pertains not alone to our science and art, but to the very hopes and fears which make us men. In seeking absolute truth we aim at the unattainable, and must be content with finding broken portions" (p. 7). A recent restatement of this concurrent need for investigation and caring can be found in Thomas' response (1976) to criticism of the medical establishment in Illich's book *Medical Nemesis*

(1976). In response to Illich's suggestion that medicine has been taken over by an uncaring scientific technology that has already reached its limits of helpfulness, Thomas replies: "Compared with the rest of biology, or with the harder physical sciences, medicine is still largely a pre-Darwin, pre-Newton enterprise. We have *not* learned everything. There is nothing like a unifying theory we can work with. The early and astonishing insight into the phenomenon of infection cannot be extrapolated to other diseases about which we are still almost *totally* ignorant. We do not yet understand the underlying mechanisms of the major illnesses which plague humanity, and therefore much of what is done in the treatment of illness must still be empirical, trial-and-error therapy. We are compelled by our limitations to resort to shoring things up, applying halfway technology, trying to fix things after the fact." Therefore, the search for specific etiologies and therapies for schizophrenia must continue, but in the meantime we have to care for individuals with schizophrenia and attempt to ameliorate the disruptions to their families and communities as best we can using the knowledge available.

Schizophrenia is a public health problem of immense proportions. It is a chronic, frequently lifetime affliction that usually begins early in life. A variety of studies have shown that between 0.25 and 0.5 percent of the United States population are currently being treated for schizophrenia, and about one percent suffer from this illness during their lifetime (Babigian 1975). That is, an estimated two million Americans have schizophrenia today, and about one million receive some sort of treatment. Schizophrenics occupy between a third and a half of all mental hospital beds, and they utilize between 10 and 18 percent of all outpatient services. The National Institute of Mental Health estimates that the direct and indirect costs of schizophrenia are about fourteen billion dollars a year. This illness is not only a disruptive and costly disease; it is also a mortal one. Studies in Monroe County, New York, found that the age-adjusted mortality rate for schizophrenics was almost twice that of the general population (Babigian and Odoroff 1969). Winokur and his colleagues, in their thirty-to-forty year follow-up of the Iowa 500 group, found that 10 percent of the 170 schizophrenics in their study had committed suicide, as compared to 10.6 percent of the depressed patients, 8.5 percent of the manics, and none of their controls (Winokur and Tsuang 1975).

Schizophrenia is also a public health issue because its treatment, especially after the first relapse, has largely been shunned by the private sector and, in the vast majority of cases, been left to public delivery systems. While some patients who have a single acute schizophrenic episode get better with or without drugs, for the majority of schizophrenic patients relapses are the rule and the illness is chronic. For these patients, public treatment is usually the only treatment because of the vast expense over a long period of time, the lack of available insurance, and, as we must acknowledge, some professional antipathy. We always suggest to first-year psychiatric residents that they follow at least one schizophrenic patient during their entire three years of training. This longitudinal experience allows them to see beyond the almost magical reintegration on the inpatient ward, to the periodic exacerbations that characterize the natural history of this disease. Many in psychiatry erroneously term schizophrenics "treatment failures" when they relapse. Operating under such a premise, the therapist often feels frustrated and ungratified in his work with them, and this feeling, unfortunately, often prompts him to relegate their care to others. As a profession we have to reevaluate our expectations and criteria for success and failure with this chronic disease and remember another medical dictum: the physician can cure few, relieve many, but should comfort most.

Deinstitutionalization

Until the 1960s, most schizophrenics were treated in mental hospitals, usually for very long periods of time and quite frequently for a lifetime. In the 1950s we became aware that the expectations inherent in the custodial environment of the state hospital seemed to foster an additional disability, which was called by a variety of names: hospitalism, institutionalism, social breakdown syndrome (Levy and Blachly 1965). Some attempts were begun to inhibit this superimposed disability by changing the values and expectations of schizophrenics within the hospital milieu through intensive rehabilitation and educative efforts. Cumming and Cumming, in their influential book *Ego and Milieu* (1962), discussed ways of reversing those aspects of the state hospital setting that promote the atrophy of ego functions necessary for living outside the hospital. Hollingshead and Redlich (1958) demonstrated that mental illness is correlated with socioeconomic class and that psychiatric services were maldistributed by both class and severity of illness.

By the early 1960s the optimistic movement toward greater social justice in many areas of our national life, as expressed by civil rights legislation, the Peace Corps, and so on, also included a demand for more equitable availability of mental health services and consequently fostered the community mental health movement (Rubin 1969). Launched by President Kennedy (1963), the movement had the distinct purpose of relinking hospitalized patients with their families and their communities in order to avoid reliance on custodial hospitals. During this same period, the improvement in our psychiatric technology, and especially the advent of psychoactive drugs, helped us see that psychotic behavior could be treated without physical restraint and perhaps did not require long hospitalization.

Several studies also showed that patients who previously would have been hospitalized for long periods of time could do just as well or better with brief hospitalization, day hospitalization, or in some cases without any hospitalization if intensive follow-up and family care were available. One of the earliest of these was the classic study "Schizophrenics in the Community" by Pasamanick, Scarpitti, and Dinitz (1967), undertaken between 1961 and 1964. The authors explored the question of whether schizophrenics could be treated at home with minimal psychiatric professional input and with minimal facilities. They randomly assigned schizophrenics who were about to be admitted to a state hospital to one of three groups: (1) a hospital control group who were admitted as they would have been without a study; (2) a group who received home care with a nonactive placebo of a psychoactive drug; and (3) a group who received home care and an active neuroleptic agent, chlorpromazine. The home care consisted of regular visits by public health nurses, who were backed up by a psychiatrist. At the end of a follow-up period, which ranged from six to thirty months, they found that the group who received home care with an active drug had the least time in the hospital, the fewest readmissions, and the greatest improvement in psychological tests, mental status, domestic functioning, and social participation. Seventy-seven percent of those people who had home care and drugs were out of the hospital during the entire follow-up period, while only thirty-four percent of the people with home care and placebo stayed out of the hospital. Families of the people on home care with drugs acknowledged that it was a burden to have these people at home but that it was worth it.

In the 1970s an added impetus for treating schizophrenics in the community has come from the courts, which have recently ruled that states cannot keep patients in hospitals without providing them with active treatment. In a recent class action suit against St. Elizabeth's Hospital in Washington, D.C., the federal district court ruled that patients are guaranteed "suitable care and treatment under the least restrictive conditions," which includes placement in community-based facilities (*Dixon* v. *Weinberger* 1974). Unfortunately, instead of prodding the states to provide an active treatment milieu within their mental hospitals, such rulings have often resulted in many state hospitals' simply emptying their wards onto the community. A public policy of "deinstitutionalization" was adopted—a password that stands for the phasing out of state hospitals as their censuses decrease and as the use of the hospitals for long-term treatment of acute episodes becomes less frequent. Ideally, deinstitutionalization would decrease the disabilities of ego atrophy and institutional dependency which were typical in custodial state hospitals and would shift the focus of care to the community. This hope had great appeal to both liberals, who were very much against the evils of the custodial state hospital, and conservatives, who saw it as a way to close state hospitals and decrease public expenditures and taxes.

What has happened, regrettably, has been anything but ideal. In many areas there has been indiscriminate deinstitutionalization without the provision of adequate services for the patients. Such indiscriminate deinstitutionalization has poisoned public opinion about the feasibility of community care, as patients have been literally dumped on unready families and into unready and unwilling communities. Arnhoff (1975), Rieder (1974), Robbins and Robbins (1974), and several others have detailed some of the disastrous effects of this violation of medicine's cardinal rule, *primum non nocere,* first do not harm. Deinstitutionalization will only work if it is followed by another neologism (one of my own coining), "recommunitization," that is, integrating patients back into a meaningful community existence at least as good as that given up by leaving the hospital.

The well-publicized woes of Long Beach, Long Island, demonstrate that indiscriminate deinstitutionalization without reintegration of patients into the community can cause significant community backlash against the mentally ill (Shapiro 1976). This community of thirty thousand, which has four percent of Nassau County's population, found itself with one third of the chronically ill deinstitutionalized patients from the whole county, over five hundred patients. Most of these people lived on welfare in delapidated hotels with little supervision or supportive services. The city reacted defensively with legal measures, trying to fend off what they saw as a horde of intruders. They tried to sue the state to provide adequate services for these people and then passed an ordinance banning further chronically ill persons from their city. Although this ordinance has since been overturned, the community climate in Long Beach certainly does not make it a very pleasant place for an ex-patient to live. As the *New York Times* editorialized, "what kind of a crusade is it to condemn sick and fearful people to shift for themselves in an often hostile world, to drag out a hungry, derelict existence in a broken down hotel if they are lucky, victimized if they are not by greedy operators of so called half-way houses that are sad travesties of a fine concept" (April 8, 1974).

In a review of what has gone wrong with deinstitutionalization, Kirk and Terrien (1975) report that the formerly hospitalized patient on the whole has not been rehabilitated, has not been reintegrated into the community, has not saved the community any money, and has not benefited from continuity of care. The authors argue that patients have not been rehabilitated because of the paucity of therapeutic living facilities and lack of suitable financial, social, and vocational services available to them. Also, caregiving staff who treat patients in the community have often themselves been transferred from state hospitals and have frequently brought along with them the hospital environment and its attitude of hopelessness. The patients have not been integrated in the community because they have usually been placed in the more deteriorated sections, the only parts of the community where people with illness would be accepted in large numbers. Kirk and Therrien cite California financial data to show that it costs more to provide good services to schizophrenic patients in a community than in a state hospital. Finally, there is little continuity of care because mental health professionals still view these patients as undesirables and offer inadequate outreach services to insure follow up; also, after evicting patients from the total care environment of the hospital, community-based care is often fragmented and provided by a variety of competing welfare, mental health, and health agencies.

A final stroke on this bleak picture is the follow-up to Pasmanick's "Schizophrenics in the Community" study, described above—in itself a classic example of what can happen if resources are not available. The grant that had funded this study ended after the third year (1964), and as a result the pilot program was abandoned, the home care with active drugs, which had proved to be so effective for two and a half years, was stopped, and the patients were left to seek help by themselves at state hospitals or outpatient clinics. Five years after the end of the program (1969) the original investigators again checked the status of these three groups of patients. They found there were no longer any significant differences in rehospitalization rate (about sixty percent of all the patients had been rehospitalized), and there were no longer any significant differences in psychological test scores, vocational functioning, or domestic or interpersonal performance (all three groups had deteriorated). The investigators found that after the home care program ended in 1964, the patient had to rely exclusively on his own initiative in fighting his way through the bureaucracy and getting the medications and care he needed. They found that throughout the three groups the patients who did best were distinguished by being married, by having gone to an outpatient clinic, and by taking their medication. The investigators concluded that the laissez-faire model of care for schizophrenics just does not work and that we need an aggressive delivery system to see that medications are taken, to support the patient and his family, and to continue the expectation that the patient will be able to function and perform tasks. In the forward to their new book reporting this follow-up study, quite aptly entitled *Schizophrenics in the New Custodial Community* (Davis et al. 1974), the authors ask themselves and their readers very serious questions "about the social implications of science, the expenditure of funds and personnel on research whose results are not utilized, and all the personal frustration of investigators who must feel the tremendous anger of what are, fundamentally, wasted professional lives . . . Can we proceed when we are aware that significant positive findings and the knowledge gained will not be put to use?" (p. xii).

Which Schizophrenics Should Be Treated in the Community

Despite the bleak picture painted so far, we wish to discuss some ways we can use the little that we do know to best serve schizophrenics in the community. First, we must decide which schizophrenics to treat in the community. This cannot be done by administrative pronouncement or professional enthusiasm but must be based on the individual evaluation of each patient's current symptoms and social skills, as well as the resources available to him within the community; that is, we must determine if he can live in the community, what types of supports are needed, and what the human and monetary costs are. We must determine if the patient's symptomatic behavior is likely to be too disruptive in a noninstitutional setting. Lamb and Goertzel (1972) have warned that we are deceiving ourselves to think that we can phase out all mental hospitals because there are always going to be some violent, incontinent, and sexually inappropriate patients who are going to need a mental institution to survive. We have to determine if the patients have or can gain, prior to their community placement, sufficient social skills to make the transfer less isolating than a hospital. Can they shop? Can they cook? Can they dress? Can they perform the basic social and interpersonal ameneties so that they do not further isolate themselves? We are not doing socially deteriorated patients a favor by asking them to cope with chaotic or disruptive neighborhoods; we certainly do not want to create more victims.

For patients who have retained or relearned basic social skills, we next have to determine what social supports in the community are available to them. Does the patient still have family or friends? Does returning the patient to the location from which he or she was hospitalized make sense for this individual? For some people who have been in the hospital for long periods of time, return to the community from which they came prior to hospitalization may not be a return to the familiar. The lack of a supportive social network frequently predates hospitalization of the schizophrenic; a patient who was first hospitalized because he was found in a disorganized state at the train station and who is later returned to his "catchment area" will not magically find a family or even a familiar conductor waiting for him. Are the necessary caring services to help the person function available? Is there a viable living situation? Are there ego-stretching activities? Is there medical and mental health care? We too often forget that a total care institution cannot be replaced solely by mental health outpatient care. Finally, we have to determine if the patient and his family want the patient to leave the hospital. We would not make the decision solely on this basis, but we should at least be courteous enough to ask, since they will be crucial in determining the success of community-based care.

Preparing Patients to Return to the Community

Schizophrenics are exquisitely vulnerable to change. Leaving the hospital is a major change for the chronic schizophrenic; for the patient who has been acutely psychotic it is a return to an environment in which he recently became upset and disorganized. Therefore, we need to prepare the patient for the change to the community while he is still in the hospital. Unfortunately, a patient is often given a new therapist, a new medication regime, and a new type of therapy, day treatment, at the same time that he is discharged from the hospital. To avoid the still too frequent loss of follow-up that occurs at this crucial transition point, we should start many of the outpatient follow-up services in the hospital. We should introduce the patient to his outpatient therapist and let a therapeutic alliance develop while the patient is still in the protected atmosphere of the hospital. Day treatment and the posthospital medication regimen can also be started in the hospital, to decrease the number of disruptive changes coincident with discharge.

It is also very helpful to have specific caregivers responsible for facilitating this boundary crossing from the hospital to an optimal setting in the community. Prior to discharge, such people, variously called expediters or interface workers (Hansell et al. 1968; Cohen 1974), can help the patient rehearse, in both words and action, the changes he will be going through. They can take the patient out to visit the home, to visit the halfway house, to see what the day treatment center is like, to figure out the logistics of how to get from their room in the community to the outpatient clinic so that appointments are kept, and so on. They can discuss the meaning of these changes with the patient and help prepare relatives, roommates, or whoever is going to be living with the patient by answering some of their questions about what to expect, how to act, and where help is available if there is a problem.

Which Services Are Necessary in the Community

From their studies, Davis, Dinitz, and Pasamanick (1974) have defined four basic types of needs that should be filled for schizophrenics living in the community. These are medications, the minimal necessities of life (food, housing, and mental health care), an opportunity to meaningfully occupy time, and social supportive services to patients' families.

Medication
A large number of studies show that patients with the disease and disability of schizophrenia do better in the community—that is, survive longer without relapse and readmission—when they are psychoactively medicated. Davis (1975) recently reviewed twenty-four controlled studies on the use of maintenance antipsychotics in schizophrenia. He found that sixty-five percent of the 1,068 patients on placebo relapsed, while only thirty percent of the 2,127 patients on active drugs relapsed. A major study by Hogarty and his colleagues of three clinics in Baltimore looked at the effects and interactions of both medication maintenance and sociotherapy on 374 schizophrenics discharged from state hospitals (Hogerty, Goldberg, and Schooler 1974a; 1974b). They

found that with or without psychosocial therapy, chlorpromazine was significantly more effective than placebo in forestalling relapse. In the two years of follow-up reported to date, eighty percent of the placebo patients had relapsed (mean relapse time being in the tenth month), while only forty-eight percent of the drug-treated patients had relapsed (mean relapse time, when it happened, being in the seventeenth month). The message here is clear: neuroleptic drugs are an essential part of a continuing treatment program for schizophrenics in the community.

We have to realize that it is harder in the community than in the more supervised hospital setting to ensure that the patient obtains his medications and takes them with reasonable regularity. For the patient to get his medications he has to have a continued relationship with the medication provider. Therefore, we have to have a delivery system with continuity of care and outreach capability to ensure that the patient does not get lost to follow-up. We have to have a care system that can contact the patient when he fails a medication appointment, that can, if necessary, visit him in his home, and that can provide ongoing care that the patient will want to stay in, so that the crucial linkage between patient and medication provider is maintained. We also must be certain that a patient who is dispensed medications takes them. This is especially a problem with the disorganized, paranoid, or angry patient. Certainly the injectable depot medications, the enanthates and decanoates, have been demonstrated to provide a greater certainty that the patient in the community is receiving the effects (and side effects) of psychoactive drugs for two to three weeks. This decreases our reliance on repeated patient compliance in an unsupervised milieu, decreases the possible stigma of taking pills in the work or social situation (although this can also be eliminated by using evening doses), but it does add a needle to the interaction, which frightens some people into avoiding their appointments. For all the medication issues, it is very important to gain the support and understanding of the family or companion of the patient. Many times we have seen friends and families talk patients into taking medications and out of taking them. To increase compliance, the patient and his family must have a clear understanding of the drug effects and side effects and a designated caregiver to discuss these with.

Policy issues concern the possible use of psychoactive medications in excessive amounts and for repressive purposes. It is frequently said that we are an overmedicated society. Unfortunately, it is true that in some settings medication for chronic patients, specifically schizophrenics, are prescribed "by the bushel." To provide quality care, clinical and administrative policies must emphasize the need to evaluate the patient frequently enough to ensure that he is on a true minimal maintenance dose and to monitor him for tardive dyskinesia and other side effects. Public policy issues include questions such as how much should the caregiver do to coax (force?) a patient to remain on medications? Should the caregiver let the patient allow himself to become psychotic by stopping his own medication? The issue of "psychiatric oppression" is frequently raised in the media. When is a caregiver, especially a public one, encroaching on an individual's rights? Does one have a right to be psychotic? These are public policy issues about which the profession can speak but which the larger society will ultimately have to decide.

Minimal Necessities of Life

Obtaining and maintaining the basic subsistence needs of food, housing, and mental health care are a problem for many schizophrenic patients, especially those who are desocialized and frightened and who have been returned to communities where there are no longer any significant others to help. Schizophrenics are often not aware of, or not able to manage, the very complex bureaucracy and paperwork which is necessary if they are to have their basic needs met in most communities. Many physicians and other providers know how hard it is, using all of their professional clout, to tangle with the huge list of public agencies that must be gone through to get someone basic living needs. How many times is one left hanging on the phone for fifteen minutes and then cut off while trying to talk to someone about welfare benefits? Consider how much more difficult it is for a disorganized, desocialized schizophrenic patient to try to cope with this bureaucratic maze; often they cannot. Therefore, the mental health delivery system has to be ready to help patients acquire the supports they need in the community.

Many schizophrenics need help in getting financial support,

since most do not have marketable skills when they are discharged from the hospital and need money either to buy their own roof and food or, if they have a family, to help their family reinclude them.

Some schizophrenic patients cannot or should not live on their own or with their families, and this necessitates a need for so-called "transitional living facilities," which include night hospitals, halfway houses, foster homes, co-op apartments, and other types of communal living arrangements. Nursing homes, which have been successfully used in many areas to deal with older, senile patients who have been in mental hospitals, usually are frightened of schizophrenics and are not amenable to being long-term living facilities. Transitional living facilities should provide more than just a roof; they can also provide graded responsibilities, group affiliation, and some level of therapeutic supervision. In order to house a lot of schizophrenics together one must determine the critical mass of patients, the critical mix of problems, and the stimulation level necessary to inhibit social withdrawal while avoiding disruptive overstimulation. Staff of transitional living facilities vary from full-time, live-in house managers to periodic visitors. However frequently they come, staff should work with patients to increase their living skills and to mediate the interpersonal difficulties that often arise in group living situations involving people with limited interpersonal skills.

There are community issues that center on such living facilities. An influx of schizophrenic patients, especially if some are highly visible or disruptive, can create community backlash. Our experience has been that it is fairly easy to convince citizens that they should support co-op apartments, both because co-ops involve a small number of patients and because they often house patients already living in the community. However, discussion of a halfway house, which would house a larger number of patients, frightens citizens because they fear it might draw additional disturbed persons to their community. Most citizens think that it is a good idea to have a halfway house in the community; few want it on their block. Fears persists that the mentally ill will cause violence and disruption of community life. We therefore have to take all appropriate measures to avoid validating these fears by making sure that we do not prematurely discharge violent or disruptive patients. We have to work with consumer boards to educate the community in order to get citizen participation and sanction for these living facilities. Enlightened citizens are the best lobbyists for the mentally ill; as professionals, we are seen both as having a vested interest in the mentally ill and as putting a burden on members of the community that we, who do not live there, will not have to shoulder. Citizens will listen to their neighbors from the community who have experiences similar to their own and yet are not fearful of patients.

In addition to community issues, there are both scientific and public policy issues that center on the question of what community living facilities are necessary and who will pay for them. A recent report of halfway houses in Massachusetts stated that ninty-four percent of the residents had a stay of less than one year, and sixty-seven percent returned to a home in the community. Such reports suggest that community living facilities for the mentally ill are truly transitional. Great Britain, by contrast, has had considerably more experience in this area. Researchers there are finding that many schizophrenics need more than just transitional facilities. A recent study by Hewitt and Ryan (1975) of ninety patients in London, seventy-seven percent of whom were schizophrenic, examined the theory that the rehabilitation process begun in the hospital can be completed in a prescribed period of time in a halfway house and that there can be a continual flow of patients from hospital to halfway house and then out into the community. They found that not only was there a small number of severely disturbed patients who had lengthy stays in halfway houses but there was also a much larger number of relatively well-functioning schizophrenic patients who stayed for long periods in halfway houses. These people were often working, taking their medications, and having few major symptoms. The authors reported that the relatively well-functioning group found the halfway house a social environment that helped maintain them at their current plateau of recovery. The living facility staff provided many things that families would normally provide; for example, the staff would make sure that medications were given, they would wake patients up in the morning to make sure they got to work, and they would be interested in the patients and what they were doing. There were also economic incentives to staying in a halfway house. Given the small amount of money these people earned, the only alternative living situation was in an isolated room. Hewitt and Ryan conclude that halfway houses should be considered part of the long-term treatment of schizophrenia in the community rather than as only transitional facilities, and that their long-term use does not signify failed rehabilitation because they provide a social environment that helps maintain a high level of functioning.

Schizophrenics in the community also need mental health care. Since we are ostensibly moving them out of the state hospital because it is custodial rather than treatment-oriented, we want to avoid offering mental health services that shift them into a new custodial community. We have to link the patients to therapeutic care in the community not only to make sure they receive their maintenance medications but also to help them develop the autonomy and coping skills necessary to deal with the stresses of community life.

Several studies have shown that schizophrenics are especially vulnerable to crises, to losses, and even to the small insults of everyday life. A recent study by Swartzburg and Schwartz (1976) reported their five year experience with 576 schizophrenic patients seen at the Brief Treatment Unit of the Connecticut Mental Health Center. The authors report that ordinary life stresses, without any clear-cut crises, were usually enough to disrupt the schizophrenics' adjustment in the community; they were then sent to the treatment unit with presenting symptoms of mild depression, marital conflict, anxiety, or some cognitive dysfunction. Swartzburg and Schwartz found that sixty percent of these patients could be treated briefly with medication readjustment and support.

Birley and Brown (1970) in London have investigated the concept of major life changes in schizophrenics prior to the precipitation or relapse of symptoms. They found a marked excess of important life changes in the three weeks prior to the onset of either the initial episode or the relapse episode in schizophrenics. The excess was noted when compared to the number of major changes in the patients' lives four-to-six weeks prior to the episode and when compared to a group of nonschizophrenic working persons of the same age. Almost half the schizophrenics experienced at least one major life change that was totally beyond their control in the three weeks prior to admission (for example, a burglary in their home, the severe illness or death of a loved one); this type of uncontrollable event had not happened to them in the previous three-week period and happened to a much lower percentage of the working comparison group. They also made the interesting finding that those schizophrenic patients who had reduced or stopped their phenothiazines in the weeks before relapse did not have more life crises during that period than the comparison group. Leff and his colleagues (1973), following up this last point, found that eighty-nine percent of schizophrenics in the community who relapsed while on active medications had major life crises in the five weeks prior to admission, while only thirty-one percent of schizophrenics who relapsed on placebo had such major life crises. They felt that a major crisis was not necessary to cause relapse in the latter group, who relapsed simply as a result of the everyday stresses of social interaction because they were not buffered by medications.

A variety of behavioral, psychotherapeutic, and social role interventions have been utilized in an attempt to help patients learn to cope with both the major crises and the minor stresses of everyday life in the community. The study by Hogarty and colleagues (1974a; 1974b) compared nonrelapsed patients who received psychosocial therapy to those who did not, and found that maximum restorative benefits require both maintenance phenothiazines and reality-oriented, problem-solving psychosocial treatment. This positive interaction of drugs and sociotherapy took from eighteen to twenty-four months to become apparent, however. This finding points out the necessity of continuing the problem-solving psychosocial therapy with the schizophrenic over a long period of time in order to have a substantial effect—a regimen not frequently undertaken. The authors conclude that "the medication clinic that simply offers pills will do little to improve the adjustment of patients beyond forestalling relapse. Those that offer psychosocial treatments exclusively will neither prevent relapse to any extent nor improve adjustment" (p. 615).

A specific therapeutic modality used with schizophrenics in the community on either a transitional or long-term basis is day treatment. Patients live in the community and come during the day (two to five times a week, for two to six hours a day) to interact in a treatment setting that provides supervision, medication, and group support and teaches certain social and living skills. In Boston, the Stepping Stone program of the Erich Lindemann Mental Health Center's Freedom Trail Clinic offers excellent day treatment, with a variety of group and individual therapeutic opportunities. There are "feelings groups" to learn how to express one's thoughts and feelings effectively to important others in the community such as roommates and family. There are also practical activities groups, such as cooking groups, budgeting groups, transportation groups, that focus on helping these people cope in the community. Medications and living situations are individually monitored within the day treatment program and outreach efforts are coordinated with day treatment staff. The program also works with and supports patients' families in a variety of ways, not the least of which is giving them a respite from the patient for several hours each week, during which they do not have to be the sole focus of the patient's dependency.

Many policy issues concerning mental health care of schizophrenics in the community are still unresolved. One of the most pressing is the confusion about fiscal and service responsibility for such patients. Rieder (1974) notes that before deinstitutionalization, state funding for the chronically mentally ill was clearly inadequate; the abysmal conditions in state hospitals were directly observable and the hospital or the state was held accountable. He says that with deinstitutionalization, funds are still inadequate, the conditions are not better, but the responsibility for patient care has become so diffuse that no one can be blamed. In addition, many community mental health programs have focused their resources on the less severely ill and have avoided taking the responsibility of providing services for schizophrenic patients discharged from state hospitals. To attempt to remedy this, Public Law 94-63, the Community Mental Health Act of 1975, mandates that posthospital care and transitional living facilities are essential services for community mental health centers and that these centers are responsible for coordinating financial, housing, mental health, and medical care. A policy issue on both a local and national level is to determine

what percentage of the limited community mental health resources and services should go to the care of the chronically ill. It
is very expensive to give these people good care, and a center
could devote its entire staff effort to this reasonably small cadre
of patients, leaving few or no resources to help people with less
serious illnesses.

The deployment of personnel and monetary resources raises
another policy issue. If we hope to get noncustodial care in the
community, the people who are chosen to treat schizophrenics in
the community should probably be different people than those
who were used to providing a custodial environment in a state
hospital, or should at least have different attitudes and expectations. We also have to recognize that extra caregivers at extra cost
will be required if we are to both maintain needed hospitals and
build better community services. Many hospitals have found that
as they decrease the patient census, the staff-to-patient ratio approaches a therapeutic level for the first time. The hospitals are
then understandably reticent to send their personnel into the
community if the result is a return to a custodial level of staffing
in the hospital.

Another policy question is whether intensive community services and insistence on therapy are socializing schizophrenic
patients into an iatrogenic debilitating sick role similar to hospitalism—a kind of "communitism." Dr. Waxler's finding (1977)
that schizophrenics in less developed countries do better in the
long run than do schizophrenics in our society might lead one to
hypothesize that in those less developed countries there are
more natural and familial, rather than public, support systems for
the mentally ill. There may also be less focus on being a "functioning," "productive" member of society in order not to be
considered sick; that is, other cultures may have acceptable non-
productive social roles that are not available in our very industrialized, work-ethic society. Short of changing our societal norms to
provide extended families and natural support systems that can
accept nonproductivity, professional caregivers to help patients
function to their capacity will probably be necessary and helpful.

Meaningful Use of Time
Psychosocial therapy, recreational and occupational therapies,
and day treatment all can help provide patients with ways to fill

their time meaningfully through participation in special group activities and "normal" activities within the community, school, and so on. However, since we do live in a work-oriented society, vocational rehabilitation services are important to help the schizophrenic gain or regain productive, esteem-providing, and possibly remunerative work. Sheltered workshops can be either an important transitional step to regain work and interpersonal skills on the way to competitive employment or may simply be a very important, long-term part of a therapeutic maintenance environment. The public policy issue is that there are not enough sheltered workshops at the moment of either kind; especially lacking are those long-term sheltered work environments for patients who are not going to be able to get into the competitive job market but for whom it is very important to have some way to maintain esteem through the useful occupation of their time.

Supportive Services for Patients' Families
There has been much controversy about keeping schizophrenic patients with their families to avoid hospitalization or returning patients to their families after hospitalization. Some studies have shown that the schizophrenic patients can often do as well at home as in the hospital if their families are well supported by mental health caregivers. Langsley and colleagues (1971) have reported an eighteen-month follow-up of three hundred patients between 1964 and 1969 who were all judged to be in immediate need of psychiatric hospitalization at the University of Colorado (the percentage of schizophrenics in this particular population is not given). Of these patients, those who had families and who lived within an hour of Denver were randomly assigned to two groups: half of them were admitted to the hospital, as they all would have been without the study, and the other half were sent home and treated by family crisis therapy teams. After eighteen-months, those patients who had not been admitted had less rehospitalization, were slightly more improved in social relations and social productivity, and were better able to handle the everyday crises of life than those who were hospitalized.

Herz, Endicott, and Spitzer (1975) found that patients (sixty-five percent of whom were schizophrenic) living with their families in the New York City area could be hospitalized briefly, the mean hospitalization time being eleven days, and have the same substantial improvement in psychopathology and same amount of readmissions as patients hospitalized for a mean of sixty days. They also found that those people, again all with families, who were briefly hospitalized were able to resume their jobs much sooner. They conclude that their study does not support either of two conflicting but popular hypotheses: first, that patients resolve acute symptoms faster if removed from the stressful life situation that may have been associated with the development of their present illness; and second, that patients recover faster if quickly released from the regressive hospital environment.

Of course, living with schizophrenic patients affects the family as well as the patient. The British studies by Grad and Sainsbury (1968) have pointed out the significant burden on families of having to live with impaired schizophrenic patients. Grad and Sainsbury report that this burden is especially felt in the acute stages of illness of patients who are treated at home as opposed to being put in the hospital, but that the burden seems to even out over the long term. They conclude that there is a need to provide significant supportive services to the family if a schizophrenic is to be treated in the home.

A recent fascinating article by Creer and Wing (1975) describes what it is like to live with a schizophrenic relative. They interviewed eighty families in Great Britain who had schizophrenic family members living in their homes, to try to understand both the patients' behaviors and the relatives' coping skills. Two primary types of patient behaviors disturbed the families. First were social withdrawal behaviors, including diminished interpersonal interaction, slowness at tasks, lack of conversation, few interests, and self-neglect. A much lesser amount of obvious disturbed or socially embarrassing behavior was also reported, such as restlessness, pacing, delusions, patients talking to themselves, and odd posturing. The relatives reported almost no violence or threats of violence; in fact, most patients were described as very timid.

The relatives' reactions included frequent bouts of anxiety that were often linked to not knowing what the patient was going to do next; depression and guilt at failing to be more helpful to the patient; a feeling in some that they were to blame for the patient's illness; frequent anger; and a lot of frustration. Creer and Wing felt that these were very appropriate responses to the behaviors of these patients. Although the relatives wanted advice on how to handle the day-to-day living situation—how much to encourage socialization, how to deal with withdrawal—most had worked out nonintrusive ways to cope with their schizophrenic relative. For a patient who was neglecting himself, not changing his clothes or taking a bath, one relative successfully intervened by laying out clean clothes and clean towels on the patient's bed. Many families had worked out acceptable alternatives to some very distressing behaviors. For example, for a patient who would get up and pace around the house all night, keeping the entire family awake, it was suggested that he might go down the block and pace in the school yard. He was able to pace, the family did not have to try to prohibit pacing, and the family was able to sleep and therefore lead a more normal life. The authors found that relatives remembered and valued professionals who had given them information and who had been interested in their plight.

Generally, the relatives felt that they needed more support in the management of these patients, and they wanted to be included in the medical and mental health planning for them. The authors conclude that by providing what we already do know—explaining medications, discussing how to provide the proper stimulation to prevent either withdrawal or relapse—and by being more available to relatives, we can be very helpful to them directly and help them be helpful to their patient relatives.

There are also studies in the British literature, by Brown, Birley, and Wing (1972), about schizophrenics who leave the hospital and come home to environments where the relatives are very emotionally expressive and demanding. These patients have a higher rate of relapse than patients that come home to cooler, slightly more distant families. Vaughn and Leff (1976) replicated Birley and Wing's study and found that a combination of maintenance medication therapy and a reduction of face-to-face contact with highly emotional or critical relatives could prevent relapse in nearly every case. They agreed that professionals can be quite helpful by being available to families in crisis, by finding other resources for the patient that will give the family some respite so that they are not the patient's total social environment, and by working with families as treatment collaborators.

Unfortunately, we do not yet have the crucial long-term studies on the effects on a child's development of living with a schizophrenic parent. Such experiments might usefully compare children growing up with two parents, one of whom is schizophrenic, to children growing up with one nonschizophrenic parent after the schizophrenic parent is hospitalized, in order to determine which course of action is best for the child.

Schizophrenia is a significant personal, family, community, and public health problem. The current trend to treat schizophrenics in the community, with or without a brief recompensating hospitalization, has obvious advantages and disadvantages. We desperately need long-term studies to understand the effects on the patient, his family, and his community of this shift of treatment to the community setting. In the meantime, physicians and mental health professionals must strive to integrate care for the schizophrenic patient and to avoid the nemesis of a new type of custodial care.

DISCUSSION

How can private practitioners work with the community mental health system? Most of us agree that it is important to have one person follow a schizophrenic patient through the treatment. So often patients, especially in public hospitals, are handled by teams instead of individual therapists.

It would be nice if there were one therapist who could follow a patient for a lifetime. It would be good for the patient and perhaps even good for the caregiver. That is, however, going to be a most rare case in the public sector. Caregivers do not, in fact, stay in the public sector very long; if they do, it is usually because they are moving away from patient care and into administration. We talk about fostering institutional transference rather than transference to a transient individual caregiver. Still, at all times there should be one primary caregiver to whom the schizophrenic relates and through whom all the other multiple caregiving resources are channeled.

How the private practitioner can work with community mental health practitioners and facilities is a major issue. Nonphysician mental health caregivers, who provide most of the services to schizophrenics in the community, have felt both intimidated and disdained by private psychiatrists, and there has been too little collaboration between the two groups in urban areas. Private practitioners have been integrated most fruitfully with community mental health in rural areas, where there is a very limited number of caregivers and no room for competition. In an urban area there are usually two systems of care, and the relationship between the private sector and the public sector is usually not very good. It is quite possible for a private practitioner to continue the psychotherapy of a schizophrenic patient and have the patient involved in a public-sector day treatment program or in a variety of other types of care in the public sector. When they can work well together, and spend the time necessary to coordinate their treatment plans, this arrangement is to the advantage of both caregivers and the patient.

Is the goal of eliminating state hospitals close to realization?
Probably not. We try to sell deinstitutionalization as being less expensive, but if done well it will be more expensive in direct, publicly visible costs. It may end up at some point as less expensive in total cost, but that is going to take a long time to prove. We always talk in extremes: total deinstitutionalization, meaning the elimination of all the hospitals, versus long-term hospitalization for all schizophrenic patients. In fact, there are many patients who feel that the quality of their lives is better in the community than in the hospital; on the other hand, there are many others who do better in the hospital. If the extreme goal of total deinstitutionalization is realized, eventually legal suits will probably be filed to get the patient back into active treatment in the hospital. We now have legal rulings that say if the state does not provide active treatment in the hospital, it must let patients out; there may soon be a suit arguing that if the state does not have active treatment in the community, it must let a patient back into the hospital.

Is there a difference between treatment techniques that are intended to prevent chronicity following an acute episode and techniques that are intended to rehabilitate the patient who is already chronic? We still have a large residual group of people whose acute episodes were twenty or thirty years ago and who have since become chronic. Is deinstitutionalization appropriate to them?
There are a few controlled studies of the rehabilitation of chronic patients. If these individuals can improve their social skills, they may be able to survive in the community. Again, the issue should not be an ideological one of whether patients should live in the hospital or in the community; rather, each individual's deficits and skills should be evaluated to determine the most appropriate living situation for that person.

Why is so little attention paid to primary prevention while so much is made of dealing with the results of devastating mental illness?
We do not know enough about etiology, and one cannot prevent something one does not understand. But while investigators are trying to understand the primary etiology of schizophrenia, we cannot ignore secondary and tertiary care. Primary prevention has been effective in the

case of certain nutritional and chemical psychoses. Personally, I have some reservations about putting most of our money into the chronically ill. Still, the problem is how can we humanely care for chronically ill patients and yet have some money left over to deal with prevention and less severe illnesses.

Would you comment on what a political football this issue of deinstitutionalization has become? Why do the politicians not listen to psychiatrists and researchers?

Scientific opinion has probably never had much influence in the public sphere. But in this case private medicine and psychiatry have basically abrogated their responsibilities to a large number of very sick patients in public institutions. These institutions attempt to take care of such patients as economically and humanely as possible, but they have rarely succeeded. Since we as a profession have never elected to treat this group of patients, they have become a public problem, and politicians, after all, are the spokesmen for the public. Some of us study schizophrenia, but few of us treat schizophrenics in the state hospital or community. So we are not in a position to complain. If we want to get back into it, there is a lot of room and work for psychiatrists in treating the chronic schizophrenic. But for many years we chose to leave the arena, and it has been taken over by others.

REFERENCES

Arnoff, F. N. 1975. Social consequences of policy toward mental illness. *Science* 188:1277–1281.

Babigian, H. M. 1975. Schizophrenia: epidemiology. In *Comprehensive textbook of psychiatry*, vol. 2, ed. A. M. Freedman, H. I. Kaplan, and B. J. Sadock. Baltimore: Williams and Wilkins.

Babigian, H. M., and C. L. Odoroff. 1969. The mortality experience of a population with psychiatric illness. *American Journal of Psychiatry* 126:470.

Birley, J., and G. W. Brown. 1970. Crises and life changes preceding the onset of relapse of acute schizophrenia: clinical aspects. *British Journal of Psychiatry* 116:327–333.

Brown, G. W., J. C. Birley, and J. K. Wing. 1972. Influence of family life on the course of schizophrenic disorders: a replication. *British Journal of Psychiatry* 121:241–258.

Cohen, R. E. 1974. Interface teams as an integrating agent in mental health services. *International Journal of Mental Health* 3:67–76.

Community Mental Health Centers Act, Public Law 94-63, Title III, July 29, 1975.

Creer, C., and J. K. Wing. 1975. Living with a schizophrenic patient. *British Journal of Hospital Medicine* July:73–82.

Cumming, E., and J. Cumming. 1962. *Ego and milieu*. New York: Atherton Press.

Davis, A., S. Dinitz, and B. Pasamanick. 1974. *Schizophrenics in the new custodial community*. Ohio: Ohio State University Press.

Davis, J. M. 1975. Overview: maintenance therapy in psychiatry, part 1: Schizophrenia. *American Journal of Psychiatry* 132:1237–1245.

Dixon v. Weinberger. February 14, 1974. No. 74285 CDDDC, District Court Case in Washington, D.C.

Grad, J., and P. Sainsbury. 1968. The effects that patients have on their families in a community care and a control psychiatric service—a two-year follow up. *British Journal of Psychiatry* 114:265.

Hansell, N., M. Wodarczyk, and H. M. Visotsky. 1968. The mental health expediter. *Archives of General Psychiatry* 18:392–399.

Herz, M., J. Endicott, and R. L. Spitzer. 1975. Brief hospitalization of patients with families: initial results. *American Journal of Psychiatry* 132:413–418.

Hewitt, S., and P. Ryan. 1975. Alternatives to living in psychiatric hospitals—a pilot study. *British Journal of Medicine* 14:65–70.

Hogarty, G. E., S. C. Goldberg, and N. R. Schooler, 1974a. Drugs and sociotherapy in the aftercare of schizophrenic patients, part 2. *Archives of General Psychiatry* 31:603–608.

––––––. 1974b. Drugs and sociotherapy in the aftercare of schizophrenic patients, part 3. *Archives of General Psychiatry* 31:609–618.

Hollingshead, A. B., and F. C. Redlich. 1958. *Social class and mental illness*. New York: Wiley.

Illich, I. 1976. *Medical nemesis: the expropriation of health*. New York: Pantheon.

Kennedy, J. F. 1963. Message from the President of the United States relative to mental illness and mental retardation. Document 58, 86th Congress, February.

Kirk, S. A., and M. E. Therrien. 1975. Community mental health myths and the fate of former hospitalized patients. *Psychiatry* 38:209–217.

Lamb, H. R., and V. Goertzel. 1972. The demise of the state hospital—a premature obituary. *Archives of General Psychiatry* 26:489–495.

Langsley, D. G., P. Machotka, and K. Flomenhaft. 1971. Avoiding mental hospital admission: a follow up study. *American Journal of Psychiatry* 127:1391.

Leff, J. P., S. R. Hirsch, and R. Gaind. 1973. Life events and maintenance therapy in schizophrenic relapse. *British Journal of Psychiatry* 123:659–660.

Levy, L., and R. Blachly. 1965. Counteracting hospital habituation. *Mental Hospitals* 16:114–116.

New York Times editorial, April 8, 1974, p. 34.

Osler, Sir William. 1922. *Aequanimitas*. Philadelphia: Blaksiton's Son and Co.

Pasamanick, B., F. R. Scarpitti, and S. Dinitz. 1967. *Schizophrenics in the community.* New York, Appleton-Century-Crofts.

Rieder, R. O. 1974. Hospitals, patients and politics. *Schizophrenic Bulletin* 11:9–15.

Robbins, E., and L. Robbins. 1974. Charge to the community: some early effects of a state hospital system's change of policy. *American Journal of Psychiatry* 131:641–645.

Rubin, B. 1969. Community psychiatry: an evolutionary change in medical psychology in the United States. *Archives of General Psychiatry* 20:497–507.

Shapiro, R. 1976. Providing care for former institutional patients puts challenge on psychiatrists. *Clinical Psychiatry News* 4:1.

Swartzburg, M., and A. Schwartz. 1976. A five-year study on brief hospitalization. *American Journal of Psychiatry* 133:922–924.

Thomas, L. 1976. Rx for Illich. *New York Review of Books* 23:3–4.

Vaughn, C. E., and J. P. Leff. 1976. The influence of family and social factors on the course of psychiatric illness. *British Journal of Psychiatry* 129:125–137.

Waxler, N. E. 1977. Is mental illness cured in traditional societies? A theoretical analysis. *Culture, Medicine, and Psychiatry* 1:233–253.

Winokur, G., and M. Tsuang. 1975. The Iowa 500: suicide in mania, depression and schizophrenia. *American Journal of Psychiatry* 132:650–651.

9

Psychotherapy

DANIEL P. SCHWARTZ

This chapter concerns the psychoanalytic psychotherapy of schizophrenia. It leans heavily on the work of many others, some of whom I will cite throughout the chapter. The bias is, however, my responsibility. It is best that I state its dimensions at the outset.

In general, I am among those who are interested in developing a psychoanalytic concept of "action." This concept of action must be one which is in concordance with the available psychoanalytic data both about human development and the processes of psychotherapeutic treatment (Hartman 1964).

More specifically, my bias is that such an action concept and its language are implicit in the problems of ego psychology, are enmeshed in much of Freud's and our own work, and are central to the articulation of any full understanding of human value and human growth. This is most clearly and notably addressed in the work of Erik Erikson (1964b).

Finally, it is my conviction that elements of this "action" concept and language can be seen and described particularly clearly in psychotherapeutic work with schizophrenic patients.

Faced with the presence of terror in the person who is undergoing a schizophrenic regression, we have learned to act. We do not blanch too quickly at the young man who says, "I have no self. Things look flat and gray. I am responsible for an evil change in this community—I must act soon or friends and teachers for whom I care will be destroyed." Frequently aided by drugs, supported by mental health centers in the community, we move to protect that person, help them manage—abate their acute regressive disorganization. As psychotherapists, our task is clear. We pursue relentlessly with that patient those interventions which are antiregressive in nature (Schwartz 1975). We search for and name the precipitating event. We gather the family or primary group together whenever possible. In occasionally tactless communication, we demand that they and the patient communicate, with a focus on or about our best hypothesis as to what has disturbed the patient and/or family's previously workable equilibrium. We support reestablishment of their previous modes of adaptive function and relation. Whenever possible we avoid a distorting intimacy and dependency upon therapeutic staff. We aggressively oppose all forms of withdrawal. We are vigorously interested in the rapidity of inner organization and the return to ordinary outer function; with the return of adaptive capacity, the person is then encouraged to pursue further psychological care of either supportive or investigative character (Gill 1954).

And all of this works and is helpful: the patient feels better, organizes, returns to his prior function and relatedness. Our antiregressive actions, our steadfast psychotherapeutic push toward organization, toward adaptive functioning, toward the reestablishment of previously operative intrapsychic and interpersonal bonds wherever tolerable, are used by that patient and often the people in his environment to recover his and their own functional capacity, to dissipate this regressive episode.

For many people afflicted with a regressive experience of a schizophrenic nature, however, no such clarity of direction exists. Neither their intrapsychic organization nor their developmental necessities nor the possibilities of their invested environment will permit those options for actions, those organizations of perception and interpersonal bonds that will facilitate in response to the usual psychotherapeutic efforts a resumption of inner organization and outer vital function. Their regression persists or they narrow their life's dimensions lest they trip into a recurrent regressive abyss. Like it or not, they sometimes do trip again, and they do this in the face of our best and most sensitive antiregressive maneuvers, the employment of useful drugs and of helpful and various family, individual, and community supportive therapeutic activities (May 1976).

One has seen all this as a psychotherapist. And when such a repetitively troubled person comes into one's presence and says, "It scares me, coming to talk with you, you know; I think, or know, that part of me is crazy—that it, that part, may grow bigger if we talk—that I may in some way die"; when the person says, "There may be only a shell of me, and if we talk and look I may find nothing in the center," one's chill as a psychotherapist is real: for the therapist and for them there is a risk (Frosch 1957).

Awe for those risks, and respect for the pains of engagement, is also acknowledged by psychotherapists upon seeing in their own hospital a person undergoing a variant of catatonic schizophrenic frenzy—a person who, having been through other short-term hospitals and left by other therapists, is writhing in restraints, mute, incontinent, panic-stricken, and disorganized.

Wisdom often dictates that, faced with such risks, one respect a patient's constricted life and help him as best one can to step around that "crazy part" a little better and help him to slowly and carefully watch the areas of safe function. Similarly, therapeutic responsibility for the risks with that frenzied catatonic patient may make one weigh one's own resources of time and energy for investment—one's own capacity as a therapist for continuity—in the balance with what one can, however dimly, gather about that person's once existing function, his lost friends, developmental organization, and briefly glimpsed environmental options. For some of us as therapists and with some patients that regressive risk is measured and met, and both decide that the probabilities, the necessity of a "valued life," demand a way out of that constriction or frenzy which involves growth, and that the risk is part of the territory.

And so therapists opt for, at least at times, a partially different psychotherapy—one that has its stake in the evolution of the valued self, in the evolution of directions of development from within the patient, in a search for a capacity to function that wrests some response, some satisfaction for the patient from himself and his environment. And in the course of that evolution therapists will deal, as best they can, with the regressive disorganization that *may* occur, deal with it in such a way as to best limit its destructiveness, sometimes its pain, but without prejudicing its utility, its part in the process of growth.

It is to aspects of this process—which psychoanalysis and psychoanalytic psychotherapy from Freud (1954) to Sullivan (1962), from Abraham (1949) to Fromm-Reichmann (1954) and Will (1961a; 1961b), from Searles (1965a; 1965b) to Semrad (1969), have engaged in courageously—that I will address myself. Since it *is* risky and involves pain, why do therapists do it? Why do the patients pursue it? Perhaps a glimpse at the experience itself will inform us. Here is a fragment of such work, of such an experience —a portion of an hour with a patient who is most often determinedly suicidal, periodically hallucinates voices demanding that she kill herself, is at times delusionally certain that I, her psychotherapist, am out to kill her.

"You are unreal," this young and troubled woman says to me, acid in her voice. "You don't exist. I can't stand your dead feel, your fishy eyes, your calculator mind. How can it be that I choose you as the person about whom I care?" She says, "Other doctors seem to be interested in me. They tell me about themselves, how they feel—they prefer me in some way. Yet I think that makes me uneasy. They like me too much. I'm too important. I don't trust it or them."

"That is an angry pain, finding me such an unfeeling person," I say.

"It seems unfair," she tells me. The inequity of it all particularly disturbs her. She thinks of me often outside our hours, and it is long from one appointment to the next. I, she imagines, think of her only when I am in her presence. Perhaps she disappears from me when she leaves the hour.

It is, I remind her, not so many months ago that she thought of herself as "unreal," the way she now thinks of me. *She* then was all intellect, cold, felt dead, and wished to die. It was as if the wind whistled through her. *She* had no substance then, I say.

She nods and pauses and in a soft voice says, "I was thinking of a movie I saw—pictures of a male seahorse having babies—the eggs, a million glistening small editions of himself come from his pouch into the water all around. It was beautiful." She looks at me as if from far away and says, "You know, only a few survive."

There is for each therapist in such experiences a seductive

beauty—a beauty in that intensity, in that rage which etches death's closeness and life's fragility in poetic conjunction (Eissler 1952). But I think that what commands and binds these two people is the possibility, in image and interactive process, of being part of, and curious observer to, the evolution of a person's sense of self.

I want to describe some regular facets of this risky endeavor—this psychoanalytically guided psychotherapeutic search for growth. One facet is best called boldly "heroic," and the other, its adjacent surface, withering "contempt." I will follow this with an attempt to understand grief's central place in growth processes where psychotherapy works. I will then note the place of exits, including termination as an exit from, a limit of, this interaction. Finally, I will include some remarks on why therapists should not be afraid of the immortal nature of images.

First the heroic. It is the case, looked at from the outside, that well-known therapists of severely ill schizophrenic patients are, in anecdote, in their own and others' writings, in common talk, all viewed in a heroic mode. Fromm-Reichmann (1950), for example, when greeted with fecal smearing by her patient, does not turn away but simply wears old clothes. Robert Knight (1946) is a giant who brooks no wavering will in his patients. Sullivan (1962) is relentlessly truthful with his schizophrenics. Will (1961a; 1961b) has a quality of indestructible presence that is available by day or night. Searles (1965a; 1965b) can tolerate within himself feelings and fantasies of extraordinary range and then put those to use in the therapeutic task. Fleck (Lidz et al. 1965) is intuitive and understanding in a manner that defies belief.

Examples abound. It was my privilege some years ago to accompany Dr. Fleck, then director of the Yale Psychiatric Institute, on his weekly rounds. He knew all the patients, their development, family structure, and so on in meticulous detail. His rounds expressed in part his medical discipline and tradition and also his regular inquiring care for the patients' welfare. During one of these tours we entered the room of a young woman who had been in the hospital for a considerable period of time. The patient greeted us with a barrage of disorganized comments—half-word salad, it seemed—about the window, her teddy bear, the bureau, the floor, dirt, the clouds in the sky, and more. Fleck listened, fixed her with a firm stare and said, "Young lady, you need to find out who you are!" The patient suddenly began to speak English. She described in clear sentences how she confused herself with the bed, her teddy bear, the clouds. As we walked out of her room and down the hall, Fleck turned to me and said, "You know, it was the damnedest thing—for a time I couldn't remember her name!"

Why is this, what is its import? Well, of course, these therapists are truly extraordinary and talented people, but we hold them in emblematic vision as heroic because they bring together that sought-for extreme of human therapeutic reactiveness that provides for and limits, as necessary, action systems—which probably all personal growth requires and which the demands of growth from a position of schizophrenic regression highlight in clarifying extremity (Erikson 1964a; 1964b).

A therapist sitting with a mute patient is suddenly assaulted by that patient, and after the mélée is handled and mutual physical security restored, the therapist is searching within himself and with the patient for aspects of his unwitting behavior that may have been a part of that occurrence. Was he, the therapist, in fact being seductive? Or was he present but not authentically responsive? Or was he too intrusive? What was the patient's own experience which precipitated and allowed that violation of their joint endeavor, that assault? Did he, the patient, become anxious? What made him so? What was involved in *his* taking the brakes off his restraint? Such honesty, I think, is heroic in its regular searching attempt.

And this sought-for honesty, this heroic integrity, curiosity, and capacity to invest are among those necessary and regular action systems that we note in the process of the psychotherapy of schizophrenia. These permit and limit the exercise of actions between patient and therapist which we call by the intrapsychic name "ego function" but which in fact include various complicated acts whose regular behavioral elaboration are vital for growth. These include actions which perceive, locate (in space and time), sequence, note similarity and difference between the person's self and others, evaluate, modulate affect and expressiveness, conceptualize, and value (Hartman 1939).

Again, what we call heroic are those actions which facilitate the conjunction of interaction of a number of conditions necessary for growth in the face of forces that would ordinarily disrupt such interaction. The management of these destructive forces involves pain on the part of both people, therapist and patient; the quality of the pain borne by the patient or therapist and their capacity to relate it and represent its relation to their joint task are elements of this activity.

Patient and therapist master the pain differently—not equally but relatedly. Patience, that old-fashioned virtue, is often brought to heroic proportions in the psychotherapy of growth from a schizophrenic position. Patience is of course displayed and demanded every day in ordinary life situations—by mothers most notably, in their developmental relationship to their young and growing children. Motherhood's special patience is, I think, also a truly heroic position—rather currently demeaned, I think, by some of our culture's other purposes, even some of those purposes which support various aspects of changing and valued development of women's growth.

But painful patience takes its shape as a therapist begins to meet that mute, frozen catatonic state with a person in a schizophrenic position. Watch them both—she a patient, he a therapist. It is not effortless for that psychotherapist as they meet hour after hour regularly, tactfully, responsively trying to decipher a word. Week after week she stands frozen, posturing, grimacing, answering no questions. She utters no words. He sits there. More weeks pass. And then she mumbles a barely audible request to her therapist: he should "abandon her, send her away, destroy her, put her to death." And the glacial grimace of her features slowly molds itself, changes to a look of more modulated, fixed despair—staring out the window. The therapist's effort is measured by the almost manic excitement he experiences as he describes these words, this change of face, to his colleagues, as he wonders aloud with the patient about her possible meanings, sufferings, intents in these few phrases. *Her* effort is unmistakable in its bleak despair, in the avoiding eye. Weeks pass. Things escalate—she makes cutting gestures in front of her abdomen and through word and gesture he comes to understand that this is the umbilical cord she is attempting to cut—to her mother, to him as her mother's agent, from herself. Weeks pass and she decreases what she eats, she throws cakes her mother has sent her into the wastebasket, she says she "has no needs," she is contemptuous in mocking gesture and disdainful epithet at the "spoiled" other patients in the hospital, and, in clipped, contemptuous manner, at the therapist himself, whose contribution is "holding on too long" to the patients.

With a leer she eats a proffered jelly doughnut and in the process smears its red and powdered white contents over her face and mouth in mocking, silent pantomime of the degrading interactive greed which, in her view, her therapist is inviting her to be part of. Weeks pass as her physician stands there readily—curious, pained, fascinated as this young woman educates him about her views, her experience. Patiently he notes (and says on occasions) those simple things all mothers know: she looks different today; I wonder what has pleased her now; she seems angry at me; her eyes look lonely—was it a very empty weekend? Weeks go by; the patient says with disdain she is not "thirsty for his [her therapist's] company" and provides her own water from the fountain in the hall.

Slowly, as she painfully allows him to hold her in his accretion of knowledge of her experience of her past life, he comes to understand her experience of ignored presence, of neglect—raised in fact by maids, ignored or cared for in fact by *other* hirelings. He evolves a held image of her through such experience unwittingly imposed by her. He learns how neglect feels—she demonstrates that the window of his office is more interesting than he, her therapist. He learns to know in action how endless silence can be, how one can be so ignored, so not seen as to in moments lose one's sense of purpose, one's clarity of boundary between self and others, to doubt the nature and value of one's own worth. But that interactive evolution of image in the face of pain and patience—in the face of patient and sickening contempt—does proceed, and in time words have more room.

One day the patient pointedly yawns. She ostentatiously taps her mouth with her hand in pretended covering and in marked emphasis of her snobbish boredom, her impolitely stifled yawn. She stares out the office window, ignoring her therapist's presence, this time with regal contempt. Her therapist wonders about

her yawn, her hauteur, gets no response to his questions, and re-
members that he had seen her in the halls that morning and had
not stopped to say hello. Perhaps she had felt snubbed by him?
He says this; she seems to listen. He says that he thinks he did
not say hello to her because it might have sounded phony to her,
a brushed off, hurried greeting. She looks at him directly and
says, "Saying hello doesn't hurt—or need to be phony." He says
that he is glad to know that she feels that way about it. He has to
learn by her telling him what she thinks and feels, he says. She
then mumbles something unclear about getting fat, and sched-
uled time, and her parents' money. Her therapist says he sup-
poses she must wonder if he himself could be interested in her or
if it is just her parents' money with which he is involved? She
says nothing during this, but her eyes focus on him. Silently the
hour draws to a close. As they get up to go, she says with filled
eyes, "Could you have a poor man's cup of coffee with me, in
some remote moment of unscheduled time?" He says he would
be pleased to do that with her, and soon. Later when they have
their cup of coffee she acts for all the world, of course, as bored as
she can be.

Clarity requires that one state one's hypotheses, however partially formed. These include more than all those essential and
useful concepts of psychoanalytic theory and knowledge, such as
oral need, aggression turned against the self, individuation from
that mother so central to man's and woman's life, ego function
inundated. Clarity must also include the hypothesis that those
ordinary people—those therapists of schizophrenic patients—
are forcefully cast into an heroic mold in the psychotherapy of
those patients, a mold in which those actions which we call by
the names of human value—patience, honesty, care—are elicited from them. These actions are demanded by the patients'
evolution of crucial systems of behavior, central to the organization and exercise of those ego functions, which the growth of a
separate self and a sense of self require.

And one must add that the other side of that heroic stance is
that action and that position of contempt, disdain, and degradation that occurs in regular congruence from the patient toward the
therapist and his value stance. And that other side is the mark, is
the measure, of all those organizable aggressive forces within the

patient which would crush new and beginning action, that fragmentary, filamentous trial of a separate self (Erikson 1964a;
1964b).

I hope not to be misunderstood. I do not mean to say that a
therapist simply assumes a heroic and virtuous stance, imposes it
or teaches it to the patient, and thereby the patient grows.
Rather, the therapist, in pursuit of the task of therapeutic presence with such schizophrenic patients, is witness and participant
in the process of the evolution of the self. And this participation
has requirements that can only be defined in terms of the actions
of the therapist. These actions of the therapist are organized
around values which are required by the necessities of the patient's evolution of a self; organizations of such actions and their
involved ego functions may accurately be described as eliciting
heroic positions.

Nor do I view the patient's stance out of the context of accumulated psychoanalytic knowledge. His sense of shame *has* its
urethral components; his sense of disgust is not divorced from
anal libidinal development; his degraded self-esteem is affected
by the malfunctioning of the forces which organize an ego ideal.
But I mean to add to our notice the conviction that contempt
makes its horrendous presence known, is experienced as largely
visual, and occurs in all those occasions when a new beginning is
ventured—all those occasions where a small, fragile edge of action which might define the self is there, as separate, as a potential self. So that one's first question—which should hang in the
mind of any therapist seeing a patient who hides as if loathing
was about to explode upon the world—is, "What have you done
new lately?" Mothers, of course, seeing their wilted adolescents,
living as they do with the flack of daily growth, know this all too
well.

One would think the trouble of this evolution, this separate
growth of self once formed, would be enough. And that is right:
in a sense it is not all trouble, it has its exuberant excitement, its
beauty. One young man I watched who had newly found some
place for his loving capacities to stretch and move within the
world found too a joy within himself. With it he savored the food
he tasted, relished its preparation, and had pleasure in its various
smells for the first time in his life. Before, in his experience, eat-

ing had been a duty, to be performed as quickly and efficiently as one could so that one could proceed onto other work. Colors at this time also occupied his life. Clothes, always before disregarded, drab, and dark, began to be exchanged for coats of many colors; he wore bright sweaters of intriguing, colorful design.

But (there is a but) accompanying the achievement of the self, alternating with its pleasure, audience to its emerging pride, is a central and concomitant sorrow—a grief so inescapable, so regular, so deep and abiding as to often appear to be the main, the overriding result of this new growth. What is this, this grief? Why its crucial position? Elvin Semrad surely understood and taught its language best (1969). It is talked about in various scientific languages. "The schizophrenic patient who recovers enters into a long period of neurasthenic experience with depressive overtones," says our descriptive psychiatric language. Some of this depression is regarded as simple enough. The patient is facing the world and his problems again—and they are painful and depressing. Yet to those of us who work psychoanalytically with such patients, who watch and participate in their growth, there seem to be more complicated aspects of their depression than can be accounted for by the simple recovery from a regressive experience. In fact, it appears to one that grief occurs in various guises on the occasion of any substantial advance in growth or organization of a separate part or a sense of that patient's self. Before I illustrate that regularity of grief and note some of its properties and consequences—its attempted avoidance by vengeful organization, its intimate connection with blame and forgiveness —I want to review grief's special place in the crucial epochs of normal development.

Early on in the field of child development it was noted that the period of growth when the eight-month-old child panicked at the sudden disappearance from sight of his mother is soon replaced by his or her capacity to weep over the mother's absence and to play, as in the "Fort-Gehen" game described by Freud (1955a), repetitively with the sense of her absence in a form which helps define its limits and sustain his mastery of the organized conception of that loss. We are not surprised that the capacity to organize such an image of that treasured mother is accompanied by the more fully developed capacity to weep.

Similarly, however one regards the peculiarities of language of Melanie Klein (1932) and some of her followers, one views with respect the observations that led her to describe in small children the manner in which anxiety and its fragmented, aggressive representation is expressed by those children in the frightening view of their own unmodulated impulses. One respects the observations of the totalistic division of imagery of parts of that child's self and its investing objects into good and safe and dangerous and bad, and the fashion in which these are slowly, developmentally, nurturingly organized into a more stable system of action and representation. The valued, caring presence of that mother, called "other," and that child's noticeable potential definition of a separate self emerge in imagery acknowledging that new organization. Klein called that monumental achievement the "depressive position," and I think with good reason, if one notes that grief is the accompaniment of its achievement.

No one who has been a party to a person's adolescence—its prolonged and exciting painful attempts and successes in organizing a separate self, separate not just from their parents, not just from being a child, but from various aspects of their own former self—no one knowing that process intimately regards the grief involved as simply pathological. It is the regular accompaniment of new inner and outer psychic organization (Blos 1967).

Schizophrenic patients say this to one straight out, with some anger and some grief. One said to a therapist in a rage as they met in a family meeting, "She did it [pointing to her therapist], she did it—she's to blame—I used to be everybody—and now I am only a person." And there was grief there to be felt.

One patient, whose speech began as a mumble and progressed to talk, wrote some simple poetry and shared that writing with her therapist. One of the poems about that process goes as follows:

> I shed my armor,
> It is hard,
> Yet, I must.
>
> It is hard,
> No one knows me
> Yet, I must.

I cry in the dark,
Who knows what is inside:
I say: leave, leave myself;
Leave the skin of myself,

If I am to grow.

And this patient's tears—silent and eloquent—were companion to that growth's grief on most of those occasions during the first few years that she and her therapist regularly met.

I suppose, nonetheless, that what finally convinces the therapist of schizophrenic patients of the central place of grief is the way in which they find themselves contending with those extraordinarily costly attempts by patients to avoid its experience. Most obvious are those young people who cling to that unworkable empty relationship with their parents—filling it vainly and self-destructively with vengeance (Searles 1965b). These are the patients who destroy each beginning of their own separate accomplishment, as they begin to feel its necessary grief. Its achievement and beginning presence demonstrate to them that they alone—not their family—will ever see or feel or care about that new reality. While sick they at least had the illusion of connection with their family in their punishing power. As one watches and is a part of that patient's dilemma, it becomes clear how much developmental capacity for grief, how much valued and anchored sense of separate self one must grow if that special state of value that one calls forgiveness is to be present (Kernberg 1975).

There is another dimension of the necessary conditions for growth of a separate self, a dimension etched in panic during psychotherapeutic work with schizophrenic patients and yet such a commonplace of normal development as to appear unremarkable. This dimension is that of limits—the limits of action and interaction, specifically that portion of it that I would like to call exits.

Everybody knows about exits—in a way. In normal families provision is made for exits from the relationships with mother and father—through friends, siblings, school, in adolescence through privacy, love, and work, and finally, through marriage and even failure. All these are of course necessary and troublesome to traverse. It is largely when they are closed, unavailable in any form at crucial times, that havoc results. That child who cannot be allowed out of his mother's sight, that adolescent who cannot leave his family, that young person who cannot have a separate friend are all in trouble. And students of the psychological events which precipitate schizophrenic regression have noted that often it was the absence of exits, a sense in the person of the absence of viable options for action, that marks the occasion on which a schizophrenic regression occurs (Lidz et al. 1965).

For those who work to provide the conditions for growth out of a schizophrenic episode—psychoanalytic psychotherapists—the avenues of exit have been and are matters of major attention, though these exits, these limits of interaction, have been called by a variety of different names.

One gifted therapist leaves her office door open for many months and her patient, who in the beginning can only stay in her presence for a few moments at a time, gradually begins to be able to sit in a chair by the side of her desk and only much later closes the door. Another schedules his times with a particular patient at the end of the day so that his schedule's rigidity does not corral this young person. Another goes for walks with his patient, who seems "trapped" by being alone with him in the office. Another does not say "I'll help you" to a schizophrenic patient but rather "I am here," since the former seems to his patient to deny the patient's autonomous options for action (Pious 1961).

Frequently it is not until a therapist can and does raise the question of the advisability of stopping his own attempt at therapeutic work with a given patient that the therapist can understand that he himself has an exit—and that the patient does, too. The patient's capacity for options in action, which will secure an awareness of exit, and the therapist's capacity to permit, survive, and recognize these real capacities are defined in congruent processes.

One young paranoid schizophrenic patient's family had enmeshed him in their own seemingly endless anxiety-ridden and corrupt practices. They would pour cheap whiskey into expensive whiskey bottles in order to save for themselves, presumably, the valuable liquor and serve their family guests and business associates cheap liquor under false label. They demanded that the patient out of family loyalty learn to keep for himself, and for his father, two sets of books—one falsified for business purposes, the other for accurate records. They prohibited him from holding his own money in his own name and prohibited him from buying anything separately for himself. The patient became schizophrenically disorganized when a situation arose that seemed to him to require an action he could not take, one which would have, if pursued, exposed this byzantine-like entrapment and family network.

With some hard work, this young man recovered from this acute regression in the course of a hospitalization, and during the crucial part of this period he assaulted his therapist, who was in the employ of the hospital in which he was treated. He had had considerable difficulty establishing a therapeutic working relationship, though the therapist was in fact quite talented. It was in time arranged that the patient should have, and pay for his own with his now self-held money, a psychoanalytic psychotherapist who was not connected with the hospital. The patient himself was not at the moment ready or able to live outside the hospital. During an early interview with his "outside therapist" the patient talked some, paused, slouched in his chair, the lower part of his face largely covered with his folded hands. He stared at the therapist unblinkingly and said, "What would you do if I slugged you?" The therapist said a number of things—not all in a rush. He first said that the patient was a free agent—free not to do that—slug him. He also assured the patient that it would certainly happen only once, that is, between them. He said that he felt that he would survive the experience of being socked but that he did not care to earn his living in that fashion, and therefore if the patient slugged him, that would be the end of their therapeutic work together. Finally, the therapist suggested that he was aware, and was certain the patient was aware, that there were other options available to the patient—for example, that of putting his feeling or thought into words and understanding what it was about.

The patient relaxed visibly and then began to describe aspects of his hospital experience which were private and the conflict that privacy presented in the face of the ideology of the hospital

—as he interpreted it—that the hospital had a right to share in all of the patient's experience, with little regard for his separateness, his different goals and experience. The avenues of exit from that hospital, from other constraining networks—and from the patient's own inner conflicting wishes and needs to be helped and be allowed to go—was a large part of the subsequent therapeutic work and experience.

Often the importance of avenues of exit are discovered by seeming inadvertence, sometimes in the midst of therapeutic despair. One finds a patient relentlessly getting worse, becoming more regressed, delusional, self-destructive, and finally one says, all right, I give up, and the patient is transferred to another therapist, quits, or is hospitalized. Then, within an extraordinarily rapid time, the patient is back on his own feet, more grown-up, and functioning at a much higher level. If the therapist is fortunate, some of these patients come back to work with him, and what they say is this: "You know, I had to find out that I could leave you, I had to find out that I could put a stop to all this— even though much of it was helping me. And the only way I guess I could do it was by failing. Once I was out of here, once I had left, I was in the hospital and I could see that you *could* let me go, that there were of course other people that I could use, that I didn't even have to grow up if I didn't want to." It seems that there have to be exits—even from one's own growth—if it is to be truly one's own, and utilizable. I am describing in the language of action and its limits the conditions under which, in psychoanalytical understandings, an ego boundary is defined, its integration into the sense of a separate self, the congruent and concomitant process of evolution of an object relationship, and the corresponding formation of a representation of an image of that invested other are accomplished.

The paramount exit for psychotherapy—that special limit of action whose existence defines our whole endeavor as psychotherapy—is of course that exit called by analysts "termination" (Freud 1955b). Traversing that exit regularly involves reworking within the context of that impending exit from the therapist and the therapeutic work—feeling and articulating, examining and integrating the numerous facets of one's historic childhood, its fantasy and experience, its loves and hates, its supports and traumas.

The process of termination in psychotherapeutic work with the schizophrenic patient does not escape nor exclude these phenomena. There are, however, two aspects of that exit experience which have an extra claim upon our attention. These are the definition of the uniqueness of the therapeutic work and, secondly, the immortal images that are involved.

Mutual definition of the uniqueness of the therapeutic work involves naming the forces, the action, the real evolutions of experience within that psychotherapeutic process, its unrepeatable nature, its determined directionality, its unique accomplishments, its unreproducible functions, its special failures. This includes the definition of who did what to whom, of what work the patient did, of what work the therapist did, and what work they did together (Zetzel 1956; Greenson 1965). More than most patients, schizophrenic patients, to grow, need to notice and locate the nature and limits of their own and others' actions.

Finally, one must acknowledge in the process of that exit, particularly in the psychotherapy of schizophrenia, the fate of those immortal images of the self and of the therapist. I say immortal images with some provocative purpose. I believe as scientists, soft scientists, misled scientists perhaps, we have so tried to avoid suggestion and manipulation and magical influence as to make particularly beginning therapists unduly wary of their own real value, their own profoundly useful therapeutic influence. We have been rightly so afraid to take advantage of our patients' longing for a good father, a perfect mother, a godlike protector— so rightly afraid that we might or did distort the truth of the nature of our therapeutic influence and relationship—that we have been unduly afraid to acknowledge the lawful evolution of the patients' creation of their own valued, immortal images of themselves as unique, separate people and their concomitant and necessary image of that unique and special therapist (Freud 1958; Wexler 1952; Schwartz 1958; Loewald 1960).

And as that joint work moves toward the mutual exit of termination, what is more clearly defined and examined is the nature of that image. It must be painfully and proudly claimed by both therapist and patient, its existence inundated by the patient's rage; its grandiose distortions, its persistence and decay in the absence of the constant contact with the therapist, its magical construction, its anaclitic relationship to childhood and lost and recreated loves—all become the exit's agenda.

And with that overcrowded work must go the acknowledgment of the absolutely unique nature of each of those people, therapist and patient, in their separateness and relation and of that "operationally" (in Bridgman's sense; 1959) unduplicatable procedure called psychoanalytic psychotherapy—whose exact parallel is not to be found among the regularities of living. Pain accompanies that creation of image; a patient wrote a poem to herself and to her therapist describing some of it. It goes as follows:

> I miss you, more and more,
>   absence makes
>   a large quarried cave
>   in me,
>
> Though quarried with
>   skillful hands,
>
> To ease the sharp pain
>   of expansion.

Another patient says, "I used to hear your voice, you know—teasing me about how powerful I thought I was, or that it was right that I was noticing that a person had a body—or that it was naturally painful to notice how dumb my boss was—but now I don't. It's as if you're still there—but I'm not occupied with that. I'm wondering now how to move that project of mine—what of me and what of them is getting in its way."

"I do still think a lot about you, though. About whether I'll disappear from your mind when I leave, about whether you'll say hello on the street after we've stopped or will I be filed away for you somehow in one of those gray filing cabinets outside your waiting room."

And if one as a therapist is prepared to say, while acknowledging that patient's anger and grief at your loss, at your allowing them to exit from your life, if one can say, "Please tell me what you have noticed about how I think of you, what you think in fact my feeling and image of you is?" you will be helpfully surprised to notice how real, how unsentimentally adamant, how holdingly accurate is that patient's vision of your image of himself, which stays within him, within you, differently, behind.

The decisive products and representation of hard therapeutic work are formed from actions elaborating ego functions on the part of the patient and therapist—actions imposed by their joint task and by the necessities of the schizophrenic patient's growth of a self. Those actions and representations are emblematized by a heroic therapeutic stance which the therapeutic task imposes around unique organizations of value and by the evolved immortal imagery of self and of other which occurs in all crucial situations of the growth of the self.

So when, as will happen, some young or older person comes to you as a therapist and says, "I was thinking of finding a 'guru'— and then I remembered your voice, that time when you stopped a moment and asked how I was, and I thought—perhaps I know one—you!" When that happens, do not be afraid—ask them to come in and tell you *all* about that. You will find yourself being educated!

DISCUSSION

Perhaps one of the problems with a heroic conception of psychotherapists of schizophrenic patients is the idealization of such therapists and the consequent feeling that these therapists have a sort of privileged knowledge and sensitivity?

That is an important point. I agree that there are dangers involved in using words like "heroic." It invokes in a therapist all the grandiose and omnipotent aspects of his own development and his enduring and frustrating wishes for closure, for final understanding, for completeness in his knowledge as to the nature of the world. To view either the patient or the therapist as heroic *can* mask, can keep from mutual scrutiny and self-scrutiny all those unconscious defensive self-images of a narcissistic, grandiose, and omnipotent character. This would certainly seriously interfere with any therapy. I also think that young therapists viewing themselves as heroic may be misled into thinking that life and therapy involve some blissful unitary solutions rather than regular, to-be-confronted conflict. This can be somewhat akin to the wish for a fusion experience which many people search for in their attempt to avoid pain and conflict—such as those who take LSD or who become submissively attached to "great leaders" who they believe will solve everything for them and for the world. In those senses I agree with your point, and I have worried about how much I might mislead such a person.

But I disagree with your point in a number of ways. I regard with some awe children and their normal processes of growth. It is only the fact that we live in the middle of such processes which allows us to overlook their regular and monumental achievements. I do think that there are some things about the awesome nature of that growth which psychiatrists have left to poets too often, although within psychoanalysis "ego psychology" and child psychoanalysis have tried to correct this. Some of Eric Erikson's work attempts most clearly, I think, to find a place within human psychology for such a study of growth. Erikson (1964b) attempts to struggle with this in his article on "actuality," where he reexamines Freud's famous Dora case. Erikson raises the question of what Dora, an adolescent (that is, a young person who is growing rapidly), wanted from Freud—the question indeed which Freud asked himself. And in relation to this question Erikson struggles with the concept of values, and their place in our understanding of human growth. In the Dora case he focuses upon fidelity as a value. He struggles with fidelity's place in Dora's family life, its place in her character structure, its place in her response to psychoanalysis, and its place in Freud's own view of himself as a scientific investigator. I have tried, to relate such a value concept to ego function and to action, and to spell out what I think is involved in that which Erikson calls "mutual activation" in the article. I use a heroic position in this paper as one such value to be named and scrutinized, in its relation to action and growth.

To call attention to these processes is also to resist labeling them too simply as just, for example, "ego strengths." Terms such as ego function, when they are too simply accepted, disguise the phenomena they are intended to illuminate, and make one not look at what is involved. Ego function, for its full definition, involves many facets of the personality, not just intrapsychic organization. It involves, I think, repertoires of behavior that are learned and supported by community endeavors and behaviors imposed upon the world by the person in the evolution of the development of such integrated ego function (and perhaps even in the sustaining capacity to exercise these functions). Heroes, we know of old, are often forced into a heroic position. They usually are not trying to become heroic but rather find themselves in a position where the forces of action are such that they need to take a stand relative to a particular development, a stand in action. I think that stand is rightly called heroic, when it finds itself to be the nidus of painfully organizing growth.

Can you comment on the risks involved, on which patients you accept into psychotherapy and which you do not?

There are a myriad of variables involved, including the response to previous treatment, relationships with others, including familial relationships and their character, early environmental history, drugs, current environmental support, and other options for action.

I do think that it is a risk for both the therapist and the patient when they work together in this fashion. This is a difficult work we do. The nature of the risk to both of that work is a complicated subject. Clear study of this requires examination by therapists of their past failures, the people in whom they have facilitated regressive disorganization unhelpfully, and comparison of these failures to people with whom they have been helpful, those who have regarded their joint work together as uniquely valuable in its experience and outcome. In practice I discuss with prospective patients as best I can the risks they run. I tell them what I think the the risks are and ask them what *they* think the risks are as best they can define them. I find that this process is illuminating, and eventually it involves a mutual decision either to work together or to find some other avenue of aid for the patient other than working with me in psychotherapy. Some of these patients I decide not to work with, especially when I think I am going to arouse an unmanageable introject, or when the ego boundaries are so friable that a sense of self is likely to be lost *before* I have a chance to establish a working relationship with that person. I try to explain this to patients in their own language. It is, however, a difficult question and should be the subject of a more lengthy discussion.

When in the psychotherapy of a schizophrenic patient do you decide that you have failed?

My view is that this is not always a clearly answerable question, a fully rational decision. One cannot always tell whether one has failed or not, and often forces outside oneself determine that decision in practical terms. The extremes, of course, are the easiest to describe. There are times when it is very clear that nothing you do is useful, when this is a consistent finding and the patient helps you clarify this observation and decision—that what you do has failed with them. They make this relentlessly clear much of the time. In such instances there is often no development of a sense of shared space, no dialogue, no movement in the material, no elaboration of the historical or current or interpersonal or intrapsychic data, no workable change in the patient's behavior. And, of course, the crucial word in all of this is "workable." With some patients one can sense that one can upset them, one can facilitate a regressive movement in a variety of ways in relating to them, but there is no indication over any appreciable periods of time that any aspect of them is moving towards a position of learning or growth or helpful change. With them one acknowledges the failure, stops the work, and facilitates where possible the patient's search for another avenue of aid.

On other occasions patients touch you as a therapist—they attach themselves and do not let you go when you are about to give up. For example, you are just about to lie down and therapeutically die, about to say, "Okay, you win; your mother wins; or your introjected uncle wins; or your conscience wins; and I can't be of any aid whatsoever." And then they say something which invites your reaching, and your capacity to keep going, and later one finds that that was very useful. One patient I remember, for example, would go for many, many weeks without anything happening except her tearing up the ward and creating a variety of disturbances in the hospital. She was not saying anything in her therapy hours with me, not even a word during most of them. I would sit there during these hours and think, "What am I doing here?" I would worry about my own psychic state, about its grandiosity, its masochism, worry about my own ego boundaries, whether I could tell if there was something that she was responding to, or whether it was instead something within me that I was inventing and projecting. Thus, at times I wondered whether I was talking to myself or which of us was the more confused. Then, to my surprise, in the midst of this mute chaos she would mumble something. I remember on one particular occasion she had not spoken a word to me for what seemed an extraordinarily long time, and then she mumbled a word, "horns," during an hour. I could not figure out for the life of me what horns had to do with anything. I thought about horns to myself, and I thought about horns aloud, and I asked her about horns, and I used the word "horns" in as many ways as I could think of, including "horns of a dilemma," and so on, and she would not say a word about horns or anything else for a few weeks. Finally, during one of our therapy hours I took my dictionary down from the bookcase and looked up and read aloud from it the various definitions of the word "horns." One of them had to do with horns being used as the symbol of a cuckold, and as I read this definition she stopped looking vacant and looked focused, alert, and directly at me, and it was clear that this was it! It was as if she had said, "You finally got it, Doc." Of course, weeks and months later a whole wide range of material relating to sexuality and adultery and unfaithfulness, her hidden witness to shameful and traumatic betrayal, became available to us in words and historical perspective within her experience. But what it is that keeps one going at such times is what the patient does to keep your own interest and investment alive and to keep you working.

I think, however, that there are times when one cannot legitimately discern the outcome. There are times when there is no sense of work going on, no useful responsiveness, only painfully apparent regression, and yet the patient eventually gets better. There are other times when all of that occurs and this is not the case; the patient does not get better. What the differences are between these times is, I think, a subject needing careful study.

From your involvement in study groups on the psychotherapy of schizophrenia, you are undoubtedly only too aware of some of the re-

*search problems in the field. In light of your description of psycho-
therapy as a unique experience, do you think that psychotherapy can be
studied scientifically?*

Yes, I think it is certainly open to scientific scrutiny. I hope I used the
word "unique" in Bridgman's operational sense of that word. What I
mean to say is that the nature of the very special rules of interaction are
the *operationally unique* definition of the situation. It is much clearer in
psychoanalysis than it is in psychotherapy, but I think both involve
clearly observable and scientifically studiable phenomena. In psychoanalysis, of course, the rules are more clearly and formally defined—
rules of action, time, fee, schedule, money, silence, the couch. I think it
is this very regularity and uniqueness that ultimately provides the scientific possibility in these situations. These are orderly actions occurring
between the patient and the therapist, and I think we do keep score and
count. Somebody with a more sophisticated system than mine could also
keep score in a very useful, scientific way. By that I do not mean that this
is a mechanical, dehumanizing experience in any way.

*Some would doubt whether psychotherapy really affects the schizo-
phrenic process or whether one is not merely living through with the
patient the course of his illness.*

That is a possible position to take, but not one with which I agree. I
think that "living through" and "growing" are different psychological
experiences. I think that recovery from a regression and growth out of a
regression involve different processes. I do not regard the conditions of
growth in the schizophrenic patient as totally unique, however, for that
situation. I think that they are continuous with a lot of other situations,
including normal human growth. I do not mean that they are indistinguishable, but that they are related, though different.

The essence of a schizophrenic episode is indeed a regression in
which unconscious and primary process material become apparent and
ego boundaries and reality testing are lost. Now, I personally do not
think you get over any experience; that is, you do not simply forget or
unlearn experience. I do not think you get over learning how to ride a
bike or forget that or unlearn that. Nor do I think you unlearn the experience of how you feel during a schizophrenic regression or how you recover from one. One can observe the forces within and around the person as they act to allow a recovery from a schizophrenic regression, and
presumably differentiate some of those which involve a recovery with
growth from those which simply involve an abatement of that regression. I think one can describe a certain orderliness of those procedures, both of the recovery from the regression and of the processes involving growth. They are not always the same. I do not mean in any way
to convey a disrespect for the fact that some of the facts of that schizophrenic experience are beyond my comprehension. There are nonetheless clearly psychological ways of influencing that process, and I see no

reason to ignore those simply because bodily physiology and chemistry are involved as well.

To follow up that question for just a moment, many investigators are now taking the position that if a patient recovers from a psychotic state and becomes clearly not psychotic, one has then to assume that the person was not schizophrenic. In other words, the only unequivocal schizophrenia is that which has traditionally been called chronic process schizophrenia, which by its very definition does not resolve. Would you care to comment on this position?

I do think that there are a lot of different psychological maladies called schizophrenia. I believe in the value of current and past efforts to sort many of these different maladies out from each other. However, it seems to me to be a fallacy to define true schizophrenia as only those whom one cannot treat psychotherapeutically and then when someone comes along and helps one of these very troubled people to recover, to grow psychotherapeutically, to turn around and say, "Well, then, I won't call that real schizophrenia." That seems to me a scientific fallacy of no small dimension.

REFERENCES

Abraham, K. 1949. The Psycho-sexual differences between hysteria and dementia praecox. In *Selected papers of Karl Abraham*. London: Hogarth Press.

Blos, P. 1967. The second individuation of adolescence. *Psychoanalytic Study of the Child* 22:162–186.

Bridgman, P. W. 1959. *The way things are*. Cambridge: Harvard University Press.

Eissler, K. R. 1952. Remarks on psychoanalysis of schizophrenia. In *Psychotherapy with schizophrenics*, ed. E. D. Brodz and F. C. Redlich. New York: International Universities Press.

Erikson, E. H. 1964a. The golden rule in the light of new insight. In *Insight and responsibility*. New York: Norton.

————. 1964b. Psychological reality and historical actuality. In *Insight and responsibility*. New York: Norton.

Freud, S. 1954. Draft H paranoia. In *The origins of psychoanalysis*, ed. M. Bonaparte et al. New York: Basic Books.

————. 1955a. *Beyond the pleasure principle*. London: Hogarth Press.

————. 1955b. From the history of an infantile neurosis (1918). In *Standard edition*, vol. 17, pp. 10–11. London: Hogarth Press.

————. 1958. Observations on transference love (1915). In *Standard edition*, vol. 12, pp. 157–171. London: Hogarth Press.

Fromm-Reichmann, F. 1950. *Principles of intensive psychotherapy.* Chicago: University of Chicago Press.

———. 1954. Transference problems in schizophrenics. In *Psychoanalysis and psychotherapy,* ed. D. Bullard. Chicago: University of Chicago Press.

Frosch, J. 1957. Severe regressive states during analysis. *Journal of the American Psychoanalytic Association* 15:491–507.

Gill, M. 1954. Psychoanalysis and exploratory psychotherapy. *Journal of the American Psychoanalytic Association* 2:771–797.

Greenson, R. R. 1965. The working alliance and the transference neurosis. *Psychoanalytic Quarterly.* 34:155–181.

Hartman, H. 1939. *Ego psychology and the problem of adaptation.* New York: International Universities Press.

———. 1964. On rational and irrational action. In *Essays on ego psychology.* New York: International Universities Press.

Kernberg, O. 1975. *Borderline conditions and pathological narcissism.* New York: Jason Aronson.

Klein, M. 1932. *The psychoanalysis of children.* London: Hogarth Press.

Knight, R. P. 1946. Psychotherapy of an adolescent catatonic schizophrenia with mutism. *Psychiatry* 9:323–339.

Lidz, T., S. Fleck, and A. Cornelison. 1965. *Schizophrenia and the family.* New York: International Universities Press.

Loewald, H. 1960. On the therapeutic action of psychoanalysis. *International Journal of Psychoanalysis* 41:16–33.

May, P. 1976. Rational treatment for an irrational disorder. *The American Journal of Psychiatry* 133:1008–1012.

Pious, W. P. 1961. An hypothesis about the nature of schizophrenic behavior. In *Psychotherapy of the psychoses,* ed. A. Burton. New York: Basic Books.

Schwartz, D. 1958. The integrative effect of participation. *Psychiatry* 22:81–86.

———. 1975. Processes of psychotherapy of schizophrenia. In *Psychotherapy of schizophrenia,* ed. J. Guderson and L. Mosher. New York: Jason Aronson.

Searles, H. 1965a. Dependency processes in the psychotherapy of schizophrenia. In *Collected papers on schizophrenia.* New York: International Universities Press.

———. 1965b. The psychodynamics of vengefulness. In *Collected papers on schizophrenia.* New York: International Universities Press.

Semrad, E. V. 1969. *Teaching psychotherapy of psychotic patients.* New York: Grune and Stratton.

Sullivan, H. 1962. *Schizophrenia as a human process.* New York: Norton.

Wexler, M. 1952. The structural problem in schizophrenia. In *Psycho-*

therapy with schizophrenia, ed. E. Brody and F. C. Redbak. New York: International Universities Press.

Will, O. 1961a. Paranoid development and the concept of self. *Psychiatry* 24:74–86.

———. 1961b. Process, psychotherapy and schizophrenia. In *Psychotherapy of the psychoses,* ed. A. Burton. New York: Basic Books.

Zetzel, E. R. 1956. Current concepts of transference. *International Journal of Psychoanalysis* 37:370.

10

The Surrogate "Family," an Alternative to Hospitalization

LOREN R. MOSHER AND ALMA Z. MENN

We are going to describe the clinical aspects of Soteria House—not so much our research, since it has been extensively discussed in a number of published articles (1972–1977), but some of the ideas that came from the family study field and influenced the project's design. Family studies are still providing us with data that encourage us to continue and modify our approach. It has now been more than five years since we started Soteria House, whose name is derived from the Greek word meaning "deliverance." Someone recently remarked, "When I first heard you talk about Soteria, I could tell myself that anything you found was probably Hawthorne effect—the result of enthusiasm. But something that lasts five years and still does any good has got to be beyond the Hawthorne effect stage." Because Soteria has survived, and has dealt with about fifty clients, we are now willing to talk about it as a new type of facilitative environment, or as a new institution. Although we were not familiar with their ideas when the project started, it is along the lines of the institutions Illich (1976) and Schumacher (1973) have been talking about that today's society needs but lacks.

Our focus will be on some common sense things—not anything highly theoretical or abstract. Societies and their institutions are constantly changing—some rapidly, some very slowly. In Western industrial societies there have been major changes in the family as a social institution. In the last century the family has shifted from being a basically rural, agrarian, extended kinship

223

system to an urban, industrial, nuclear unit. Family ties are looser and less often defined by biological relationships; they are now more often motivated by mutual needs for companionship. Today's family has many nontraditional forms: communes with group child-rearing arrangements and group marriages, to cite two examples. Roughly twelve percent of families have only one parent. Last year for the first time there were more divorces than marriages.

One cannot discount these kinds of changes, and one of the jobs of mental health workers is to be leaders in changing and developing new social institutions that are responses to changing social conditions. New social institutions are needed that are more appropriate to the needs of individuals. Therefore, rather than concerning ourselves with trying to adapt individuals to existing social institutions, we as mental health workers should attempt to bring new, more relevant and appropriate social institutions into being. Psychiatry for far too long has over-invested in individual psychopathology. By the same token, it has invested too little in the processes of growth—development, change, and learning. We would do well to be more interested in learning about and helping facilitate processes of human development, not only through a focus on individuals but also through changing social conditions.

A look at medicine in general reveals a very interesting trend that we think will be magnified over the next five to ten years. More and more medicine has begun to look at ways in which environmental conditions can be modified to affect a disease or disorder. A simple example is smoking and heart disease. Doctors counsel people who have heart disease that smoking is not good for them and that they should give it up if at all possible. That advice is a simple environmental manipulation that attempts to prevent worsening of an existing medical disorder. Hypertension is another good example of a medical problem whose treatment includes a significant component of environmental manipulation. In many ways the Soteria project is designed as a psychiatric attempt to do the same sort of thing, that is, to manipulate environmental conditions to alleviate or prevent the worsening of a particular expression of human distress—schizophrenia. That *is* part and parcel of what medicine in general, and psychiatry in particular, should do and will do more and more as we begin to find out how toxins in our environment either cause or exacerbate various disorders.

Psychiatric disorders may be seen as resulting from the failure of society's institutions to respond to an individual's needs. The institutions we are talking about are the family, school, peer group, church, welfare system, and so on. Soteria is, from this perspective, an institution created to be more responsive than existing facilities seem to be to the needs of particular kinds of individuals.

We now know that certain aspects of family life are associated with the development of psychosis. At Soteria House we attempt to provide an environment within which an individual's needs can be responded to differently from the way the family was willing or able to respond. We believe this surrogate family experience is particularly important for the late adolescent–early adult group we are studying. In general, the subjects in this study are attempting to separate from their families of origin and establish themselves as separate and independent individuals. We recognize that this age group is a small segment of the total psychiatric population—but a very important one. It is young people, after all, whose lives can be severely affected over a long period of time by what is defined as psychiatric disorder. We admit only persons who are sixteen to thirty years of age in order to obtain a group whose members are more likely to be confronting the issues of independence—separation from family, proper vocational choice, education career, and mate selection. Most existing mental health institutions have not really addressed the special needs of this group adequately.

Soteria House has other criteria that must be met before an individual is accepted. We do not accept patients with extensive prior hospitalization because we feel that people who go into psychiatric hospitals learn very quickly what the role of the patient should be—how patients should act and how they can manipulate the system in order to stay in or get out. At this point we have chosen not to have to deal with the learned mental patient role. Therefore, a criterion for admission is that the subject have had no more than one previous hospitalization for two weeks or less with a diagnosis of schizophrenia.

We accept subjects of either sex, but we exclude married subjects because we believe it is important to concentrate on a group
at risk for prolonged disability. Statistically speaking, married
persons deemed schizophrenic have much better prognoses than
unmarried ones (Rosen et al. 1971).

Finally, we admit only those subjects who are clearly schizophrenic and who are considered to be in need of hospitalization.
In diagnosing the subject as schizophrenic, we require the presence of at least four of the following seven symptoms at admission and two days later:

1. Thinking or speech disturbances.
2. Catatonic motor behavior.
3. Paranoid traits (for example, systematized delusions, suspi-
   ciousness, ideas of reference).
4. Hallucinations.
5. Delusional thinking other than systemized.
6. Blunted or inappropriate emotion.
7. Disturbance of social behavior and interpersonal relations.

In addition we require one hundred percent consensus between
three independent judges (two research psychologists and one
psychiatric consultant) that the individual is schizophrenic.

Let us try to describe what Soteria is like. It is a twelve-room
house located in a suburban community in the San Francisco Bay
area. A 1915-vintage house, it has rather large rooms, including
about eight bedrooms, three common rooms, and so forth. It is
located in what is euphemistically called a transitional neighborhood, which means it is on the way down. It is a designated poverty area populated by a mixture of ex-state-hospital patients, a
small number of blacks, about twenty percent Chicanos, and
blue collar workers or college students, who make up the rest of
the population. Most residents of the area live in houses like Soteria except that they have been divided into smaller apartments.
The neighborhood also has a mixture of small businesses and a
general hospital located about a block away.

The characteristics of the Soteria environment that we think
are particularly important are shown in table 10.1. In each instance, the characteristic is contrasted with that found in the set-

Table 10.1. Comparison of the Soteria House environment to the typical community mental health ward.

Soteria House	Community mental health ward
Institutional variables	
Nonmedical	Medical
Nonhospital	Hospital
Open	Closed or restrictive
Varied work schedules	Eight-hour staff shifts
Minimal use of medication	"Usual" treatment with medication
Labeling, stigmatization minimized	Labeling, stigmatization inevitable
Behavior of residents and staff open to scrutiny and discussion	Staff behavior usually reviewed in closed sessions
Social structure	
Nonauthoritarian	Authoritarian
Nonhierarchical	Hierarchical
Peer-fraternal relationships	Parent-child relationships
Program flexibility	No program flexibility
Role differentiation minimized	Institutionalized role definitions (nurse, social worker)
"Residents"	"Patients"
Equality stressed	Patient's submission to authority stressed
Dyadic, triadic units emphasized	Group emphasized
Individuals usually responsible for and in control of their lives	Hospital, doctor, and ward assumes responsibility and control
Power resides equally in each resident and staff member	Power resides in hierarchy: head nurse, doctor, hospital administration
Minimal structured activities	Emphasis on structured activities
Continuity of relationship after discharge	Contact with hospital after discharge discouraged
Family-like atmosphere	Hotel or boardinghouse atmosphere
Family	
Vacation from psychotic offspring	Continued involvement necessary
Aftercare decided upon by individual, perhaps not involving family	Aftercare determined by doctor and usually family (if available)
Degree of involvement determined by family	Degree of involvement dictated by institutional policy.

ting where our control subjects receive their inpatient care. The characteristics that we have tried to emphasize in this special environment are relatively nonmedical. It is not a hospital; it is open; the staff do not work eight-hour shifts; and we do not very often use neuroleptic medication. We hope that by not being a hospital and by using a nonprofessional staff with minimal psychiatric input, the whole process of labeling, developing a mental patient identity, and stigmatizing will be minimized. We also like to have everyone's behavior open to scrutiny; that is, the staff are very much a part of Soteria and so their behavior is as much a part of the social system as is that of the patients. As institutions go, Soteria House is small—it only holds six patients and two staff at any one time. In that kind of setting, one can be relatively nonauthoritarian because smaller, less complex environments do not need much authoritarianism to function effectively. It can also be relatively nonhierarchical; the relationships there are more on the order of peer or fraternal relationships (staff are similar to the clients in age and background) than parent–child relationships. Role differentiation is minimized in that both staff and residents serve a variety of functions with one another. Generally, staff take on more responsibility, but there is no one staff member who is the "family therapist" or the "social worker" or whatever. Both staff members and residents do whatever needs to be done, including spending prolonged hours in one-to-one contact with very crazy people, or taking crazy people off to the dentist to have their teeth fixed, or taking them to welfare, or taking them to rehabilitation to get them into that system. If, for example, one patient has been through the social welfare system and sort of knows his way, he will take another patient with him and take him through, so that the staff does not have to do it. Everyone has a voice and shares the work, insofar as that is feasible. We believe that Soteria's size, homeyness, location in the community, and nonmedical orientation all contribute to its being less threatening to the clients because it is less discontinuous with their usual environment, as compared to a psychiatric ward in a general hospital.

We think people need a special environment to help them recover from acute psychosis. One common and important problem of acutely psychotic people is the difficulty they have in paying attention or making sense out of a complex social situation. So we try to minimize the complexity of their social interactions. Because the simplest social situation is two or maybe three people, we do not have mandatory large group meetings. We view individuals, insofar as possible, as responsible for and in control of their own lives. We do not view ourselves as being responsible for individuals unless they make it manifestly clear that they cannot assume responsibility for certain aspects of their lives. We stress that power resides relatively equally across the entire social group—although, realistically, staff views are given greater weight.

We have very few structured activities; we want to let people structure their own activities, and we help them devise whatever they want. We encourage and allow the continuity of relationships after discharge. This can mean relationships of patient to patient, patient to staff, staff to staff, or whatever combination. We try to create a home-like atmosphere; and, just as in a home, certain tasks have got to be shared and accomplished by the people who live there. We have no cook that comes in to cook the meals, there is no cleaning person who comes in to clean the floors, and so forth.

Having briefly described what Soteria is like, we would like to describe some of the family processes for which it is designed to provide a corrective, alternative, or more responsive experience. Table 10.2 identifies some family characteristics that have been described in families with psychotic relatives. In each instance, the important characteristic of the treatment setting that would tend to alleviate and ameliorate rather than reinforce those characteristics is listed next to it. Family processes are divided into three broad areas—roles, affect, and communication—in keeping with the categories used by Jacob in his recent review (1975). The listing is intended to be illustrative, not comprehensive. Readers wishing greater explication of these characteristics and comprehensive coverage of this area are referred to Jacobs' excellent review.

Clearly, staff attitudes are going to be important if a treatment setting is to provide the type of responses needed to provide this different experience for the client. Table 10.3 (again, contrasted with those found in the control setting) shows the staff attitudes

Table 10.2. Characteristic processes in families with psychotic relatives, and treatment techniques used at Soteria to offset these processes.

Family process	Treatment technique
Roles	
Stereotyped roles; invalidation; nonacknowledgment	Flexibility of response; no prescribed roles; validation; acknowledgment
Contradictory expectations	Predictability; honesty
Pseudomutuality	Flexible trial and error learning; autonomy and individual responsibility
Weak, dependent offspring used to fill parental needs; consensus sensitive; inability to affect fate	Decisions made by patient; expectations made overt; definition of needs and goals by patient; opportunity for success experiences
Symbiotic union	Continuity of relationships based on mutual consent
Affect	
Criticism; inconsistency; emotional divorce; lack of empathy	Acceptance; tolerance; warmth; support; involvement; empathy
Helplessness	Focus on patient's definition of *his* needs; help in attaining goals
Covert reject	Expression of affect
Communication	
Irrationality; unclear, vague meaning	Simple, clear, declarative, communication
Inability to share a focus of attention	Focused attention; simplified dyadic contact
Mystification	Validation of patient's perceptions of his experience

we try to reinforce at Soteria. Perhaps they can best be summarized by saying that all the troubled residents of Soteria are mentally in a very different place than the staff members are, but the staff try to do everything they can to be in that place with them. They try to share the patients' psychological space—without reinforcing it but also without trying to force them to give it

Table 10.3. Comparison of staff attitudes at Soteria House and at the typical community mental health ward.

Soteria House	Community mental health ward
Psychosis is a valid experience	Psychosis is an illness, therefore not an intimate part of the person
"Being with" the individual is important	Maintaining objectivity and distance is important
Understanding the experience is stressed	Putting the experience behind is stressed
Individual should be allowed to experience his psychosis	Individual should shore up defenses to suppress, repress, and abort psychosis
Regression is allowed	Regression is prevented or interrupted when possible
Environment stresses containing or holding	Environment stresses "moving on"
Growth and learning from psychosis is valued	Getting over psychosis quickly is valued
Pressure to "get going" is minimal	Length of stay is seen as critical

up. Staff members try to protect the patients, be with them, be real, be honest, be simple (meaning not delivering complicated interpretive statements), and to take seriously the fact that this person is in painful, traumatic life crisis. We do not believe an episode of psychosis is like getting up and shaving in the morning; it has a deep, powerful effect, more on the order of the effects of the Coconut Grove fire. The staff members take the psychosis seriously, try to pay attention, deal with it, hope that the person can get through it and not come out of it as a psychological cripple. However, we do not glorify it. Psychosis is much too painful to be glorified. It can be seen as an opportunity for change and growth without being glorified.

It may legitimately be asked, are these attitudes a *reality* at Soteria? We have used several instruments to assess independently the presence or absence of these characteristics in the environment. The one that we have used most is the Moos Ward Atmosphere Scale, a self-report, 110-item scale that measures how the respondents perceive their social environment. It has been used

COMPARISON OF STAFF AND PATIENT REAL COPES PROFILES

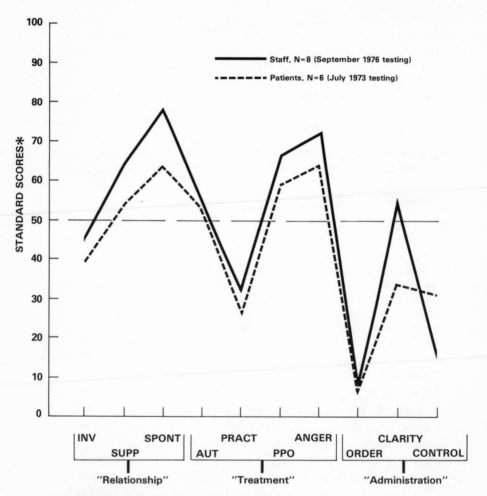

Fig. 10.1. Soteria staff and patient profiles on the Moos scale.

in all kinds of environments: psychiatric wards, halfway houses, dormitories, fraternities, and so on. Figure 10.1 shows the Soteria staff and patient profiles on the Moos scale. All scores are standard scores, so that each ten-point increment represents one standard deviation. The Soteria milieu is perceived as about the average for involvement, high on support and spontaneity, high on autonomy, low on practicality, high on person–problem orientation, high on tolerance of anger, low on order, rather low on clarity, and low on staff control. Such a pattern makes us more confident that we have, in fact, created the type of environment intended. Note also that the overall profile patterns are similar for staff and patients, indicating a congruence of views.

We think that what happens after people leave Soteria should be indicative of whether or not they were provided with a different type of family experience by their temporary surrogate family. Interestingly, a number move out as groups or in pairs to live together. As compared with our control subjects, significantly more ex-Soteria residents are living independent of their families of origin two years after admission (table 10.4). Also, they less often use halfway houses. It would seem that something about the Soteria experience does allow persons who go through

Table 10.4. Comparison of psychosocial adjustment of individuals in the experimental and control groups.

Living arrangements	Experimental group	Control group	Exact probability[a]
	Prior to admission		
	N=37	N=39	
With parents or other relatives	68%	62%	0.81
Independently[b]	30%	36%	
Board and care	3%	3%	
	Two years after admission		
	N=25	N=23	
With parents or other relatives	36%	52%	.044
Independently[b]	64%	35%	
Board and care	0	13%	
Social relationships[c] (mean ± S.D.)	1.95 ± 0.59	1.56 ± 0.92	

[a] For row-by-column contingency table.

[b] Includes living alone, with peers, or with spouse and/or children.

[c] Includes number of friends, nonfamily social visits, and participation in social organizations. Range of scores is 0 − 3.

there to disengage themselves—as is normative for their age group in this culture—from their families of origin. Thus, one of the basic aims of the project apparently is being accomplished. Brown and colleagues (1966) in England have amply documented that discharged patients not living with their families do better over the long run than those living with them.

In some ways Soteria House continues to operate as a quasi-extended surrogate family for many ex-residents while they are in the community. That is, it continues to provide names and addresses of friends, a meeting place, social activities, help with living arrangements, transportation, discussion of personal problems, and referral to various community resources.

DISCUSSION

One of the most unconventional aspects to Soteria as you describe it is the apparent tolerance of all sorts of behavior. Is there any kind of limit setting in the traditional psychiatric sense?

There is a funny story about that. We started the project with three rules: Rule 1 was that it would be made very clear that we would prevent anyone from hurting himself, hurting anyone else, or doing something that we thought would jeopardize the program. For example, undressing on the front lawn is a no-no because we know that the police would come by and that would be the end of us. Rule 2 is that we allow no tourists; that is, we do not consider Soteria to be a museum or a zoo where people can traipse through and look at the animals in the cages. Rule 3 is that Soteria obeys the laws of the land. For example, in California people over twenty-one can drink, so there is alcohol in the place; marijuana is illegal, so marijuana is not allowed in the house. Well, we had these rules, but we were also training the staff to go along with people, to be with them, even when they were quite psychotic. Two of the first three people admitted were young women who were, in the course of their madness, very hypersexualized and had the uncomfortable habit—uncomfortable for the male staff—of climbing up in the male staffpersons' laps and attempting to seduce them. Everyone got together and said, how are we going to deal with this because we are all so uncomfortable? So they devised what amounts to an incest taboo—there is to be no sexual activity between staff and clients. This rule still stands today.

Would you say more about the results of Soteria?

That is a whole topic in itself and has been published in detail elsewhere. We will just mention two findings briefly. The average length of stay at Soteria is roughly five months, while the average length of stay for our control group is twenty-eight days. The total costs for the first six months of care for the two groups are within fifty dollars of one another.

The values that you inculcate in your staff are not so different from what we all teach—openness, honesty, concern, "straight talk." I wonder why you seem to have succeeded where we often are frustrated?

Staff members often seem to get imbedded in gigantic health institutions and spend an awful lot of time with pieces of paper and meetings and talking to each other and answering queries from hospital administrators and so forth. There is a lot of value and importance in really spending time with individuals, and this is not given a high status, at least in most institutional settings. Instead, there are large hierarchies, at the bottom of which are the "mental health technicians," or whatever they are called, who are the lowest paid and least educated people. They spend the most day-to-day time with patients, yet their work is not seen as the critical ingredient in the therapeutic environment. For us, it is *the* critical ingredient. Certainly, staff are generally well-intentioned, but sometimes we can all be victims of our training. Our common sense gets trained out of us in favor of a more formal learned response to severe distress. Generally, if many staff members of big institutions were put in a place the size of Soteria, they would probably soon begin to talk and act like other Soteria staff. They would like it better themselves, and the patients would likewise come out the better for it.

To follow that issue further, there is the whole question of violence— violence among patients or between staff and patients. What do you do?

We do whatever has to be done. If someone is standing in front of the television when someone else wants to watch it, we say, would you please stand aside? If the patient turns around and starts to swing, well, the other people defend themselves or the staff members do. Or a staff member grabs and holds that person so that he or she cannot hurt or be hit. There are all kinds of ways in which the staff handle those kinds of situations. Your question may be, how often is the place not able to handle a particularly violent person? How often have we had to send patients to the regular mental health system? In five years, we have shipped out three. So obviously it is not the perfect environment, but we do pretty well.

Perhaps a more basic issue lies beneath the last two questions. How much of Soteria's success is due to the fact that in a small, intimate setting with intense staff involvement one cannot help but do much better than in a large institution? If we had the resources to divide up large state hospitals in small units with six to seven residents, would the same results occur?

We do not pretend that we are relating to the entire psychiatric population; certainly we do not want to extrapolate our data to chronic populations of state hospitals. On the other hand, a lot of what we do at Soteria could be used on many other psychiatric wards. The small size, the intimacy, the family-life orientation *is* important. One patient had come in from the emergency treatment unit and had thrown furniture around there and broken up the place. He came to Soteria and immediately quieted down and did very well. Two months later the psychiatrist who had seen him in the emergency unit asked him why he had broken up their unit and not Soteria. He said simply, "You wouldn't do that to anyone's home." That was his explanation and it is an important point. An environment like Soteria tends to elicit the best from people.

How often do you use medication?

Eight percent of the Soteria subjects have received therapeutic courses of phenothiazines. We define a therapeutic course as two or more weeks of 300 mg of Thorazine or its equivalent. For the first six weeks no subjects receive medications unless it is absolutely imperative. In the five years of the study there have been less than a dozen doses of neuroleptics given during the first six weeks.

I wonder if you would say more about how you find and train staff.

The one statistic we have not computed is the average length of stay for the staff. It has shifted over time. When we started, the average length of stay for the staff was about a year. Now, the average length of stay is probably more like two-and-a-half to three years. When we started we did a lot of intensive training of the staff. We had access to a state hospital and went on the wards there with our prospective staff members and worked with them on a one-to-one basis. The project started out very slowly; in the first year we only took in about six or eight clients because we were gradually training the staff. Now, the staff themselves train all the new staff. To get a job there you have to be a volunteer for a period of time and when the next job becomes available, the people who are living there select the new staff members from that pool of volunteers. We still do some staff training and we have a consultant psychiatrist who does a small amount of training, but most is done within the house and by the staff.

Could you place Soteria, conceptually, within the framework of the various psychiatric orientations?

The goal of Soteria is to help facilitate individual patients in finding and achieving their own goals. The "treatment" nearest to this program would probably be moral treatment. On the other hand, we are often compared to Laing's Kingsley Hall, a more "existential" conception. The major difference between Soteria and Kingsley Hall is our explicit transitional expectation. Kingsley Hall was an asylum, without any real expectations of leaving. Another important difference is that we have a paid staff and they did not.

Do you get involved in family work?

That is one of the big defects in the program. By the time people get to us, something has happened and somebody has said, "You have to go to a hospital." Ideally, we would like to be one step ahead of that and get to them before that point. We would prefer to intervene in the family system before that decision gets made and reified. Once a person is on that hospital track, it is hard to derail. We do relate to families but in very odd ways. We do not have any formal program of family therapy, but occasionally when there is a major difference of opinion, usually about where an offspring is going to go when he leaves Soteria, we will meet with families. We bring everybody in and we act as facilitators of the negotiations between the offspring and family; that could possibly be seen as family therapy. Of course, we do not have any married people, so we are not talking about relating to spouses.

Do you consider one of your goals to be like Laing's, for patients to "experience their psychosis"?

Some people who come to Soteria want nothing to do with their madness; they spend all their time running as fast as they can away from it, and that is all right. But if they feel that they in some way want to go through that process without anybody trying to abort it or force it into some pigeon hole or divert it, then we allow them to try to do this. But maybe at most sixty percent of the people who come through Soteria actually "experience their psychosis," while the others tend to run away from it.

What is your relapse rate when patients are not maintained on antipsychotic medication?

Our cumulative two-year readmission rates are sixty-seven percent for controls and fifty-three percent for Soteria-treated subjects—a nonsignificant difference. To our surprise, six weeks after admission our patients and control patients are basically indistinguishable in terms of symptoms, even though one hundred percent of the control patients have had therapeutic courses of neuroleptics and no Soteria subjects had. We did not expect symptoms to be alleviated by six weeks of interpersonal intervention. We thought it would take more like six months. Maintenance phenothiazines are a separate issue, and one which needs a lot of rethinking. Over the next several years a great deal of attention will be devoted in research to the question of maintenance phenothiazines, given the nature of their long-term toxicities. Even on maintenance phenothiazines there is still a fifty percent two-year relapse rate, whereas on placebo it is about eighty percent. So you are giving a very toxic drug to a large number of people to achieve this thirty percent additional benefit. We think that the whole question has to be reevaluated in terms of benefit versus risk. It is certainly a researchable issue.

Are your diagnoses reviewed periodically?

Initially, the diagnosis is made by the admitting psychiatrist in the emergency treatment unit. This is then reviewed by a research psychologist and a third evaluator who is a psychiatrist.We demand a one hundred percent, three-person consensus for inclusion in the study. The diagnosis is reviewed two days later. At the six-week assessment we re-diagnose, but by that point many of the subjects, because they are better, would no longer warrant the label. However, they are still in the study because we want to avoid the circularity inherent in the view that if you get better, you are not schizophrenic. So far we have had three people admitted into the study whom we subsequently had to eliminate from the research data because they were later thought to have an affective disorder.

How do you set goals with patients?

In general we expect our patients to set their own goals. Our job is to help them achieve these goals if we can, and to tell them that their goals are beyond our capacities to be of help if they are. In the second instance we would probably try to get patients to redefine their goals in such a way as to make it possible for us to help.

REFERENCES

Brown, G. W., M. Bome, B. Dalison, and J. K. Wing. 1966. *Schizophrenia and social care.* Maudsley Monograph 17. London: Oxford University Press.

Hirschfeld, R., S. Matthews, L. Mosher, and A. Menn. 1977. Being with madness: personality characteristics of three treatment staffs. *Hospital and Community psychiatry* 28:267–273.

Illich I. 1976. *Medical nemesis: the expropriation of health.* New York: Pantheon.

Jacob, T. 1975. Family interaction in disturbed and normal families: a methodological and substantive review. *Psychological Bulletin* 82:33–65.

Menn, A. Z., and L. R. Mosher. 1975. The Soteria project, an alternative to hospitalization for schizophrenics: some clinical aspects. In *Schizophrenia 75,* ed. J. Jorstad and E. Ugelstad. Oslo: Universitetsforlaget.

Mosher, L. R. 1972. A research design for evaluating a psychosocial treatment of schizophrenia. *Hospital and Community Psychiatry* 23:229–234.

Mosher, L. R., and A. Z. Menn. 1975. Soteria: an alternative to hospitalization for schizophrenia. In *Current psychiatric therapies,* vol. 15, ed. J. H. Masserman. New York: Grune and Stratton.

————. 1976a. Community residential treatment for schizophrenia.

Paper presented at the Annual Meeting of the American Psychiatric Association, Miami, Florida, May.

_____. 1976b. Dinosaur or astronaut? One-year follow-up data from the Soteria project. In *A symposium: followup studies of community care*, ed. M. Greenblatt and R. D. Budson. *American Journal of Psychiatry* 133(8):919–920.

Mosher, L. R., and A. Z. Menn. 1977. Lowered barriers in the community: the Soteria model. In *Alternatives to mental hospital treatment*, ed. L. I. Stein and M. A. Test. New York: Plenum.

Mosher, L. R., A. Z. Menn, and S. M. Matthews. 1975. Soteria: evaluation of a home-based treatment for schizophrenia. *American Journal of Orthopsychiatry* 45:455–467.

Mosher, L. R., A. Reifman, and A. Menn. 1973. Characteristics of nonprofessionals serving as primary therapists for acute schizophrenics. *Hospital and Community Psychiatry* 24:391–396.

Rosen, B., S. Klein, and R. Gittelman-Klein. 1971. The prediction of rehospitalization: the relationship between age of first psychiatric treatment contact, marital status, and premorbid asocial adjustment. *Journal of Nervous Mental Disorders* 152:17–22.

Schumacher, E. F. 1973. *Small is beautiful: economics as if people mattered*. New York: Harper and Row.

Index

Abraham, K., 200
Acetylcholine receptors, 144
Adenylate cyclase, 128
Adolescence: schizophrenia in, 84–87
Adoptees: schizophrenia in, 48–59, 64, 70n, 92
Adoptive families: mental illness in, 50–59
Adrenergic receptors, 145, 148
Affect: disturbances in, 101, 155
Alanen, Y. O., 61, 76
Almond, R., 12
γ-Aminobutyric acid activity, 148
Amphetamine-induced behavior, 123–125, 138
Angrist, B., 124
Anscombe, G. E. M., 24
Anticholinergic potency of drugs, 144, 148
Antipsychiatrists, 108
Antipsychotic drugs, 125–147, 152–167; early development of 103; molecular structures of, 125–126; behavioral effects of, 126–127; potencies of, 126, 128; effects on neurotransmitter receptors, 128–147; blocking of dopamine receptors, 138, 156; tardive dyskinesia from, 141–143, 154, 163–164; extrapyramidal syndromes from, 143–144, 155–156, 161; autonomic sympatholytic effects of, 144–145; anti-

cholinergic potency of, 144, 148; affinities for alpha and dopamine receptors, 145; contraindications for, 153–154; indications for, 154–155; types of, 156–157; metabolism of, 158; dosage of, 158–162, 165; and drug holidays during therapy, 161, 166; combined with other drugs, 162–163; sudden death from, 164; prediction of outcome with, 166–167; after discharge from hospital, 180–182; for Soteria subjects, 236, 237
Aphasia, 21–22
Apomorphine: binding to neurotransmitter receptors, 131–132; behavioral effects of, 138, 141, 143
Arieti, S., 71, 91
Arnhoff, F. N., 175
Astrachan, B., 116
Autism, 101

Babigian, H. M., 172
Baldessarini, R. J., 143
Baron, M., 65
Barrett, J., 114
Barry, H., 64
Bastian, H. C., 22n
Bateson, G., 71, 77
Benjamin, L. S., 70n
Biochemical investigations, 122–149
Biological approach to etiology, 8–9,

Biological approach to etiology (*Continued*)
15, 22–30, 104–105; historical aspects of, 99–119
Birley, J., 185, 191
Births in winter months: and schizophrenia incidence, 64
Blachly, R., 173
Blakar, R., 71
Bleuler, E., 3, 78, 100–102, 117
Bleuler, M., 13, 71, 91
Blood studies, 122
Blos, P., 208
Bockoven, J. S., 6, 8, 15
Borderline syndromes, 118
Borus, J. F., 15, 171–194
Boundary disturbances in schizophrenia, 71, 75, 76, 80, 81–82, 91
Bowers, M., 79
Braithwaite, R. B., 24n
Brentano, F., 24
Bridgman, P. W., 29n, 214
Brown, G. W., 185, 191, 234
Bunney, B. S., 127
Burnham, D., 11
Burt, D. R., 130, 136, 140, 141, 143
Butaclamol, 130–131
Butler, J., 6, 7
Butyrophenones, 147. *See also* Haloperidol

Cameron, N., 79
Carlsson, A., 127
Carpenter, W. T., 116, 118
Catatonic patients, 79
Category formation, 82, 88
Caudhill, W., 11
Chestnut Lodge, 10–11
Chisholm, R., 24
Chlorpromazine, 125; potency of, 126; binding to neurotransmitter receptors, 132; metabolism of, 158
Chlorprothixene, 156
Chromosomal abnormalities, 66
Chronic disease approach to schizophrenia, 112
Community care of patients, 171–194; and deinstitutionalization procedures, 173–178, 193; failures of, 175–177; and selection of patients for placement, 178–179; and preparation of patients, 179–180; medication in, 180–182; services necessary for, 180–192; living facilities for, 182–185; halfway houses for, 183–185; and coping with crises or stress, 185–187; psychosocial therapy in, 186; day treatment in, 187; funds for, 187–188; personnel for, 188; and sheltered workshops, 189; and supportive services for families, 189–192; private practitioners in, 192–193; as political issue, 194
Community resocialization therapy, 11–12, 16–17; in Soteria House, 17, 233–234
Comte, A., 28
Concepts of schizophrenia, 3–19
Connell, P. H., 124
Cornelison, A., 71, 72, 84
Cowie, V., 23
Creer, C., 190
Creese, I., 15, 122–149
Cumming, E., 173
Cumming, J., 173
Cummings, J. R., 130

Dalen, P., 64
Davis, A., 178, 180
Davis, J., 105, 123, 126
Day treatment programs, 187
Definitions of schizophrenia, 5, 70–71, 100, 102, 114
Deinstitutionalization of patients, 173–178, 193
Dementia praecox, 100, 101
Depression: antipsychotic drugs in, 155
Developmental theory of schizophrenia, 69–92; criticisms of, 118
Diagnosis: and labeling of patients, 108–109, 110; criteria for, 111–112, 113–114; and Present State Examination, 113, 114; new approaches to, 113–115; national differences in, 114; and Research Diagnostic Criteria, 114; and emphasis on symptoms, 114, 117; and borderline syndromes, 118
Dibenzoxazepines, 157
Dilthey, W., 33
Dimsdale, J. E., 12

Dinitz, S., 174, 180
Disease: concepts of, 99
L-Dopa, 124
Dopamine receptors: blocking of, 127–128; binding of drugs to, 130–134; antipsychotic drugs affecting, 138, 156; change in number of binding sites, 143
Dopamine system: amphetamines affecting, 124; binding to neurotransmitter receptors, 132, 134; activity in schizophrenia, 147, 148; and hypothesis of schizophrenia, 147, 156
Droysen, J. G., 28, 33
Drugs: antipsychotic, 125–147, 152–167; binding to neurotransmitter receptors, 130–136; and receptor supersensitivity, 141–143
Duhem, P., 26n
Dynamic psychiatry, 30–34
Dyskinesia, tardive, 141–143, 154, 163–164

Earle, P., 6
Eddington, A., 36
Ego boundaries, 71, 75, 76, 80, 81–82, 91
Egocentricity, 82–83; of parents of schizophrenics, 79–80; of schizophrenic patients, 79–81; in adolescence, 85, 87
Eissler, K. R., 201
Ellenberger, H. F., 31
Endicott, J., 114, 189
Enkephalin receptors, 134
Environment: and schizophrenia, 60–65; and milieu therapy, 11–12, 16–17, 223–234; and families of schizophrenics, 69–92, 229
Erikson, E., 31n, 197, 202, 206, 216
Ernst, K., 91
Esterson, A., 72
Etiology: scientific approach in, 8–9, 15, 22–30, 106–109; heredity and environment in, 47–67; developmental theory in, 69–92, 118
Existentialism, 12–13, 17–18
Extrapyramidal syndromes, 143–144, 155–156, 161

Fabraga, H., 106

Families of schizophrenic patients, 60–63, 69–92, 76–77, 229; schizophrenia incidence in, 70n; communication in, 72, 77; skewed pattern in, 74–75, 80; schismatic pattern in, 75–76, 80; supportive services for, 189–192
Family: functions in child rearing, 73; as factor in schizophrenia, 110; changing structure of, 223–224; surrogate, in Soteria House, 223–238
Family therapy, 92
Federn, P., 81
Fieghner, J. P., 113
Feyerabend, P., 40
Fischer, M., 70
Fleck, S., 71, 72, 84, 201–202
Flint, R., 24
Fluphenazine, 125; potency of, 126; binding to neurotransmitter receptors, 132; extrapyramidal side effects of, 144
Foundationalist view of science, 29
Fox R. C., 106
Frank, P., 29n
Freeman, J. M., 65
Freud, S., 31–32, 80, 89n, 200, 207, 212, 213
Friedhoff, A. J., 122
Friends Asylum, 6
Fromm-Reichmann, F., 10, 200, 201
Frosch, J., 199

Genetic factors in mental illness, 47–67, 92
Geschwind, N., 22n
Gibson, R., 11
Gill, M., 198
Gilles de la Tourette syndrome, 155
Giovacchini, P., 16
Gladstone, A., 11
Goertzel, V., 178
Goldberg, S. C., 180
Goldstein, K., 22n
Grad, J., 190
Greengard, P., 127
Greenson, R. R., 213
Grey, J., 9
Grieving in psychotherapy, 207–212
Grinker, R. R., 118

Group psychotherapy, 153
Guideau: trial of, 9
Gunderson, J., 118
Guntrip, H., 16
Guze, S., 105

Halfway houses, 183–185
Haloperidol, 125, 157; behavioral effects of, 126; effects on dopamine receptors, 128; binding to neurotransmitters, 130, 134; extrapyramidal side effects of, 144; as alpha-adrenergic blocker, 148; in Gilles de la Tourette syndrome, 155
Hansen, S., 122
Harré, H., 24
Hartford Retreat, 6
Hartman, H., 197, 202
Hatow, E., 171–194
Havens, L., 22
Health care system, 107
Hempel, K., 24n, 29n, 32
Heredity: and environment, 47–67, 70
Herz, M., 189
Heston, L., 70n
Hewitt, S., 184
Historical concepts of schizophrenia, 3–41; and biological approach, 99–119
Hogarty, G. E., 180, 186
Hollingshead, A. B., 174
Hollister, L., 15, 152–167
Home care programs, 174, 177
Hook, E. B., 23
Hospitalization: and attitudes toward treatment, 103–104; and deinstitutionalization, 173–178, 193; legal aspects of, 175, 193; surrogate family as alternative to, 223–238

Identification, 75, 76
Illich, I., 171, 223
Incidence of schizophrenia, 172; in families of patients, 70n
Individuation of child, 81, 82; parental role in, 73
Indolics, 157
Inhelder, B., 85
Insanity: definition of, 5

Intentionality, 24, 33
International Pilot Study of Schizophrenia, 113
Isoproterenol, 132
Iversen, L. L., 128

Jackson, D., 77
Jackson, J. H., 22n
Jacob, T., 229
Jacobsen, B., 54, 55
James, W., 24
Janowsky, D. S., 123
Janssen, P. A. J., 125, 126, 145
Jaspers, K., 12
Jones, Maxwell, 11–12, 16
Jung, C. G., 101

Kebabian, J. W., 128
Keller, M., 114
Kennedy, J. F., 174
Kernberg, O., 4, 209
Kessler, S., 70n
Kety, S., 15, 47–67, 70n, 92, 118, 122
Kinney, D., 63–64, 66, 67
Kirk, S. A., 176–177
Klawans, H. L., 142
Klein, D., 105, 126
Klein, M., 208
Klerman, G. L., 99–119
Knight, R., 201
Kobayashi, R. M., 141
Kohut, H., 4
Kraepelin, E., 9, 22, 25, 99–101, 117; and neo-Kraepelinian psychiatry, 22–30, 104–105, 117
Kringlen, E., 70n, 92

Labeling theorists, 108–109, 110
Laing, R. D., 17, 72, 108
Lamb, H. R., 178
Land, J. P. N., 24
Language: and explanation of disorders, 27, 35–36; patterns in families, 72, 77
Leach, E., 88
Leff, J. P., 186, 191
Legal aspects of hospitalization, 175, 193
Levy, L., 173
Lidz, R., 91

Lidz, T., 16, 60, 69–92, 201, 210
Lindqvist, J., 127
Lithium therapy, 155, 163
Living facilities for schizophrenic patients, 182–185
Loewald, H., 213
Loftin, J., 61
Lorenz, M., 90
Loxapine, 157
LSD, 135–136
Lucia, A. R., 22n

MacDougall, L., 122
Mach, E., 28
MacLean, P. D., 32n
Mahler, M., 73, 81
Manic-depressive disorders, 100, 101; antipsychotic drugs in, 155, 163
Margolis, P., 12
Maudsley Hospital, 113
Maxmen, J. S., 15
May, P., 199
May, R., 17
McConaghy, N., 78
McLean Hospital, 6
Medical model of mental illness, 8–9, 15, 22–30, 106–109; criticisms of, 108–109
Meehl, P., 78
Menn, A. Z., 223–238
Mental illness: medical model of, 8–9, 15, 22–30, 106–109; as myth, 109, 110; and schizophrenia as disease, 110–113
Mental retardation, 65, 112
Meyer, A., 10, 104
Meyer-Gross, W., 105
Milieu therapy, 11–12, 16–17; in Soteria House, 17, 223–234
Mischler, E., 116
Molindone, 157
Moos, R. H., 12
Moral treatment of patients, 6–8, 14
Mortality rate for schizophrenics, 172
Mosher, L., 17, 223–238
Mudd, S. H., 65
Munkvad, I., 124, 126
Muscarinic receptors, 144

Nagel, E., 24n

Nature–nurture interaction, 47–67
Neo-Kraepelinians, 22–30, 104–105, 117
Neuroleptics, see Antipsychotic drugs
Neurotransmitter receptors: amphetamines affecting, 124; neuroleptics affecting, 128–147; binding of drugs to, 130–136; agonist and antagonist states of, 134–135; ionic influences on, 134–135; drug-induced supersensitivity of, 141–143
New York State Psychiatric Institute, 113
Noradrenergic receptors, 144–145
Norepinephrine: amphetamines affecting activity of, 124; binding to neurotransmitter receptors, 132; intravenous, lethal effects of, 145

Objective–descriptive psychiatry, 22–30
Odoroff, C. L., 172
Organic basis of schizophrenia, 8–9, 15, 23, 106–109
Organic brain syndromes, 101; antipsychotic drugs in, 155
Osler, W., 171
Osmond, H., 15, 110
Outcome predictions: variations in, 116; and use of antipsychotic drugs, 166–167
Overinclusiveness in thought disorders, 79

Papez, J., 32
Paranoid patients, 79, 89
Parents, see Families
Parsons, T., 106
Pasamanick, B., 174, 177, 180
Peroutka, S. J., 144
Perry, T., 122
Personality analysis, see Psychotherapy
Personality development: family role in, 73
Pharmacologic agents, see Antipsychotic drugs
Phenothiazines, 125, 156; behavioral effects of, 126
Piaget, J., 79, 80, 81, 82, 85, 89n

Pieri, L., 135
Pinel, P., 6, 107
Pious, W. P., 210
Pollin, W., 70
Popper, K., 34
Preoperational children, 83
Present State Examination, 113, 114
Promazine, 125; potency of, 126; binding to neurotransmitter receptors, 132
Promethazine: potency of, 126; binding to neurotransmitter receptors, 132
Psychiatry: neo-Kraepelinian, 22–30, 104–105, 117; dynamic, 30–38; discussion of concepts in, 38–41; and views of antipsychiatrists, 108
Psychopharmacology, see Antipsychotic drugs
Psychosocial therapy, 186
Psychotherapy, 10–11, 15–16, 30–34, 153, 197–220; risks in, 199, 216–217; example of, 200; heroic aspects of, 210–206; and growth of separate self, 205–207, 209; and role of grieving, 207–212; and avenues of exit, 209–212; termination of, 212–215; and idealization of therapists, 215–216; failures in, 217–218; scientific studies of, 219; effectiveness of, 219–220

Quine, W. V., 25, 26, 39

Randrup, A., 124, 126
Rapaport, D., 31, 33
Ray, I., 6
Redlich, F. C., 174
Regression, 84, 87, 88–89, 198, 219
Rehabilitation approach in therapy, 14–15
Relatives of patients, see Families
Research: and evolution of scientific nosology, 99–119; and biochemical investigations, 122–149
Rickert, H., 33
Rieder, R. O., 175, 187
Rimmer, J., 63
Robbins, E., 175
Robbins, L., 176

Robins, E., 105
Rorschach testing of parents, 61, 62, 63
Rosen, B., 226
Rosenhan, D. L., 108, 110
Rosenthal, D., 48, 55, 70n, 91, 92
Rosman, B., 78
Roth, M., 105
Rubin, B., 174
Russell, B., 24
Ryan, P., 184

Sainsbury, P., 190
Savodnik, I., 19, 21–41
Scarpitti, F. R., 174
Scheff, T., 108, 110
Schismatic family pattern, 75–76, 80
Schizoaffective disorders, 155
Schizophrenia: definitions of, 5, 70–71, 100, 102, 114
Schooler, N. R., 180
Schuldenfrei, R., 26
Schulsinger, F., 50
Schumacher, E. F., 223
Schwartz, A., 185
Schwartz, D. P., 16, 197–220
Schwartz, M., 11
Scientific approach to psychiatric disorders, 8–9, 15, 22–30, 116–119; and neo-Kraepelinians, 22–30, 104–105, 117; and medical model of mental illness, 106–109; and schizophrenia as disease, 110–113
Searles, H., 10, 16, 200, 201, 209
Secord, P. F., 24
Seeman, P., 131
Segal, H., 16
Seigler, M., 110
Sellars, W., 28n, 29
Semrad, E. V., 200, 207
Shapiro, R., 176
Sheltered workshops, 189
Shershow, J. C., 3–19
Shopler, E., 61
Sick role, 106, 116, 188
Siegler, M., 15, 122
Singer, M., 61, 62, 71, 77, 91
Skewed family pattern, 74–75, 80
Skinner, B. F., 25, 106
Slader, E., 105

Slater, E., 23
Snyder, S. H., 122–149
Socialization of child, 73
Society: sick role in, 106, 116, 188; as factor in schizophrenia, 110, 225
Sociotherapy, 186
Solberg, H., 71
Soteria treatment treatment community, 17, 223–234; criteria for admission in, 225–226; description of, 226–229; staff attitudes in, 229–231, 235; environment created in, 229–233; ex-residents of, 233–234; rules in, 234; results of, 234–235; training of staff for, 236; medications in, 236, 237; goals of, 236, 238; family work in, 237; readmission rates in, 237; review of diagnoses in, 238
Spiroperidol, 130, 134
Spitzer, R., 105, 114, 189
Stanton, A., 11
Stebbing, L. S., 36
Strauss, J. S., 113, 116, 118
Suicide rate, 172
Sullivan, H. S., 10, 117, 200, 201
Surrogate family studies, 223–238
Swartzburg, M., 185
Sydenham, T., 99
Symptom constellation and diagnosis, 114, 117
Szasz, T., 108, 109, 110

Tardive dyskinesia, 141–143, 154, 163–164
Tarsy, D., 143
Taylor, C., 29
Tefft, H., 122
Therrien, M. E., 176–177
Thioxanthenes, 156
Thomas, L., 171, 172
Thorazine, see Chlorpromazine
Thought disorders, 70, 78–79, 89–90
Tienari, P., 70n
Tranquilizers, see Antipsychotic drugs

Treatment: historical aspects of, 6–13; psychotherapy in, 10–11, 15–16, 30–34, 153, 197–220; milieu therapy in, 11–12, 16–17, 223–234; antipsychotic drugs in, 125–147, 152–167; community issues in, 171–194
Tsuang, M., 173
Tucker, G. J., 15
Tuke, W., 6
Twin studies, 48–59

Ungerstedt, U., 141
Urine studies, 122
US–UK study of schizophrenia, 113–114
Utica Hospital, 9

Vaillant, G., 53
Van Bever, W. F., 125, 126, 145
Van Putten, T., 17
Van Winkle, E., 122
Vaughn, C. E., 191
Virchow, R., 99
Voith, K., 130
Von Hungen, K., 135
Von Wright, G. H., 33

Waxler, N., 116, 188
Weber, M., 33, 34
Wender, P., 48, 55, 62, 70n
Wexler, M., 213
WHO study of schizophrenia, 113–114
Wild, C., 78
Will, O., 200, 201
Wilson, P. T., 105
Wing, J., 113, 190, 191
Winokur, G., 105, 172, 173
Winter months: births in, 64
Woodruff, R. A., 22, 23n, 113
Worcester Hospital, 8
Workshops: sheltered, 189
Wynne, L. C., 61, 62, 71, 72, 77, 91

Zetzel, E. R., 213

CONTRIBUTORS

JONATHAN F. BORUS, M.D.
Director, Psychiatric Residency Training and Subspecialty Training in Social and Community Psychiatry, Massachusetts General Hospital
Assistant Professor of Psychiatry, Harvard Medical School

IAN CREESE, Ph.D.
Assistant Professor of Pharmacology, Johns Hopkins University School of Medicine

ELAINE HATOW, B.A.
Research Associate, Massachusetts General Hospital

LEO HOLLISTER, M.D.
Veterans Administration Hospital, Palo Alto, California
Professor of Medicine and Psychiatry, Stanford University School of Medicine

SEYMOUR S. KETY, M.D.
Director, Laboratory for Psychiatric Research, Mailman Research Center, McLean Hospital
Professor of Psychiatry, Harvard Medical School

GERALD L. KLERMAN, M.D.
Alcohol, Drug Abuse and Mental Health Administration, United States Public Health Service
Professor of Psychiatry, Harvard Medical School

THEODORE LIDZ, M.D.
Career Investigator, National Institute of Mental Health
Sterling Professor of Psychiatry, Yale University School of Medicine

ALMA Z. MENN, A.C.S.W.
Project Director, Mental Research Institute, Palo Alto, California

LOREN R. MOSHER, M.D.
Chief, Center for Studies of Schizophrenia, National Institute of Mental Health

IRWIN SAVODNIK, M.D., Ph.D.
Director, Medical Student Education in Psychiatry and Assistant Professor of Psychiatry, University of Pittsburgh School of Medicine

DANIEL P. SCHWARTZ, M.D.
Associate College Physician, Amherst College
Consultant in Psychiatry, Massachusetts General Hospital
Lecturer in Psychiatry, Harvard Medical School

JOHN C. SHERSHOW, M.D.
Director, Inpatient Psychiatric Service, Massachusetts General Hospital
Instructor in Psychiatry, Harvard Medical School

SOLOMON H. SNYDER, M.D.
Distinguished Service Professor of Psychiatry and Pharmacology, Johns Hopkins University School of Medicine